Bone Cements and Cementing Technique

Springer

*Berlin
Heidelberg
New York
Barcelona
Hong Kong
London
Milan
Paris
Singapore
Tokyo*

G. H. I. M. WALENKAMP, D. W. MURRAY (Eds.)

Bone Cements
and Cementing Technique

U. HENZE and H.-J. KOCK (Coeditors)

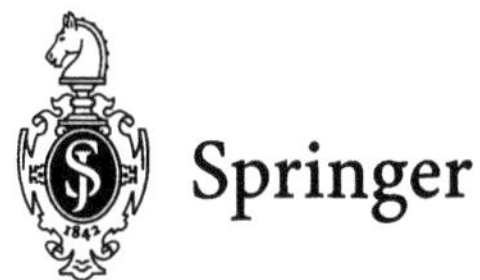

Springer

Editors

G. H. I. M. WALENKAMP
Academisch Ziekenhuis
Orthopaedie
P. Debyelaan 25
Postbus 5800
NL-6202 AZ Maastricht

D. W. MURRAY
Nuffield Orthopedic Center NHS Trust
Windmill Road, Headington
Oxford, OX3 7LD
UK

Coeditors

U. HENZE
IZKF Biomet
Technical University Aachen
Pauwelsstr. 30
D-52074 Aachen

H.-J. KOCK
Traumal Surgery
University of Essen
Hufelandstr. 55
D-45122 Essen

ISBN-13:978-3-540-41677-7   e-ISBN-13:978-3-642-59478-6
DOI: 10.1007/978-3-642-59478-6

Springer-Verlag Berlin Heidelberg New York
Library of Congress Cataloging-in-Publication Data
Bone cements and cementing technique / G. H. I. M. Walenkamp, D. W. Murray, eds. p. cm.
   Includes bibliographical references and index.
ISBN-13:978-3-540-41677-7
   1. Bone cements. 2. Bones – Surgery. 3. Orthopedic surgery – Miscellanea. I. Walenkamp,
   G. H. I. M. II. Murray, D. W.
   RD684.B655 2001   617.4'71–dc21   2001018890

Springer-Verlag Berlin Heidelberg New York
a member of BertelsmannSpringer Science+Business Media GmbH

http://www.springer.de

© Springer-Verlag Berlin Heidelberg 2001

Typesetting: K+V Fotosatz GmbH, Beerfelden
Cour design: design & production GmbH, Heidelberg
SPIN 10778841   18/3130/ag – 5 4 3 2 1 0 – Printed on acid-free paper

Contents

VI Osteolysis

Subject Index

List of Contributors

Dr. NICHOLAS A. ATHANASOU
Nuffield Orthopedic Center NHS
Trust
Windmill Road, Headington
Oxford, OX3 7LD
United Kingdom

Dr. STEFFEN J. BREUSCH
Orthopädische Universität Heidel-
berg
Schlierbacher Landstraße 200a
69118 Heidelberg
Germany

Mr. JOHN G. BROWN
Musgrave Park Hospital
Belfast BT9 7JB
Northern Ireland

GOTTFRIED H. BUCHHORN
Orthopädische Klinik
Universitätsklinik Göttingen
Robert-Koch-Str. 40
37075 Göttingen
Germany

Dr. BIRGITTE ESPEHAUG
Department of Orthopaedic Surgery
Haukeland University Hospital
5021 Bergen
Norway

Dr. WERNER EGE
Mailänderstr. 18
60598 Frankfurt
Germany

Dr. GÖTZ VON FÖRSTER
ENDO-Klinik Hamburg
Holstenstr. 2
22767 Hamburg
Germany

Dr. LARS FROMMELT
Institut für Infektiologie, klinische
Mikrobiologie und Krankenhaus-
hygiene
ENDO-Klinik Hamburg
Holstenstr. 2
22767 Hamburg
Germany

Dr. OVE FURNES
Department of Orthopaedic Surgery
Haukeland University Hospital
5021 Bergen
Norway

Dr. THORSTEN GEHRKE
ENDO-Klinik Hamburg
Holstenstr. 2
22767 Hamburg
Germany

Dr. LEIF IVAR HAVELIN
Department of Orthopaedic Surgery
Haukeland University Hospital
5021 Bergen
Norway

FRED KJELLSON
Biomaterials and Biomechanics
Laboratory
Dept of Orthopedics
Lund University Hospital
S-221 85 Lund, Sweden

Dr. HANS-JÜRGEN KOCK
Merck Biomaterial GmbH
Frankfurter Straße 250
64271 Darmstadt
Germany

Dr. KLAUS-DIETER KÜHN
Heraeus Kulzer GmbH & Co. KG
Philipp-Reis-Straße 8/13
61273 Wehrheim im Taunus
Germany

Prof. Dr. D. MURRAY
Nuffield Orthopedic Center NHS
Trust
Windmill Road, Headington
Oxford, OX3 7LD
United Kingdom

Dr. T. NORMAN
Musculoskeletal Research Center
Dept. of Mechanical & Aerospace
Engineering
and Dept. of Orthopedics
West Virginia University
P.O. Box 9196
Morgantown, WV 26506-9196
USA

Mr. ANGEL L. RUIZ
Musgrave Park Hospital
Belfast BT9 7JB
Northern Ireland

Dr. AFSIE SABOKBAR
Nuffield Orthopedic Center NHS
Trust
Windmill Road, Headington
Oxford, OX3 7LD
United Kingdom

KATRIN SCHELLING
Asterweg 7
71706 Markgröningen
Germany

Dr. RAINER SPECHT
Merck Biomaterial GmbH
Frankfurter Straße 250
64271 Darmstadt
Germany

Prof. Dr. GEERT H. I. M. WALENKAMP
Dept. Orthopaedic Surgery
Academic Hospital Maastricht
Postbox 58 00
6202 AZ Maastricht
The Netherlands

Dr. JIAN-SHENG WANG
Biomaterials and Biomechanics
Laboratory
Dept of Orthopedics
Lund University Hospital
221 85 Lund
Sweden

Prof. Dr. HANS-GEORG WILLERT
Orthopädische Klinik
Universitätsklinik Göttingen
Robert-Koch-Str. 40
37075 Göttingen
Germany

I Introduction

Introduction

G. H. I. M. WALENKAMP, D. W. MURRAY

Since the first use of bone cement, there has been much discussion about this important tool in arthroplasty. Many authors consider the cemented prosthesis as the gold standard when evaluating the outcome of primary prostheses.

In a large number of total hip arthroplasties, as registered in the Scandinavian Hip Registers, important differences in revision risks have been documented between hospitals. These differences are partly due to the use of diverse cement techniques. In the analysis of data, the influence of these techniques, as well as the different cement types, is clear.

A recent disaster with a newly developed cement also illustrated that the quality of the cement must be assured, and that the introduction of a new material must be carefully prepared and followed-up.

The new Palamed cement has been developed by the makers of the well-known Palacos and Refobacin Palacos, which appeared to be the best cements in the Swedish register. An improvement was noted in slightly better handling characteristics, but the end product is the same as Palacos. As mentioned, this cement will be carefully followed-up in the near future. However, its introduction is a good reason to gather the expertise of some of the leading figures in the field in this book.

II History of Bone Cements

Industrial Development of Bone Cement
Twenty-Five Years of Experience

W. EGE, K. D. KÜHN

Introduction

Many years of intensive research by Otto Röhm led to the development of poly(methylmethacrylate) (PMMA), the basis of bone cements, in 1934. In 1936, Kulzer was founded by the German firms Heraeus and Degussa to produce artificial dentures made from PMMA. In 1936, the cold curing of methylmethacrylate was developed in Kulzer's laboratory.

About 100 years ago, Themistokles Kluck, a German surgeon, tried artificial hip replacement. The prosthesis was made from ivory with colophony, or rosin, as glue, but that total hip replacement failed.

In 1958, Sir John Charnley [1] first succeeded in anchoring a femoral head prosthesis with PMMA cement. In 1964, Kulzer started producing and selling it under the trade name of Palacos® R. At first it was sold in bulk (1 kg of powder and 500 ml of liquid) and surgeons had to prepare the necessary portions themselves. But soon it was changed to ampule and prepackaged powder forms. Some years later, Buchholz [2] began studies on the known basis that a small amount of residual monomer is released from the bone cement. Together with the German companies Kulzer and E. Merck in Darmstadt, he initiated investigation of the addition of antibiotics to bone cements. Numerous clinical studies at the Endoklinik in Hamburg followed. As a result of this research, Kulzer and Merck developed the first antibiotic bone cement, Refobacin®-Palacos® R, which has been sold since 1972. Since then, the successful use of bone cements in orthopedic surgery has helped thousands of patients.

Methods and Results

Since the introduction of Palacos® and Refobacin®-Palacos® R, several in vitro and in vivo studies have been carried out by Kulzer and Merck to underline the excellent properties of these PMMA bone cements.

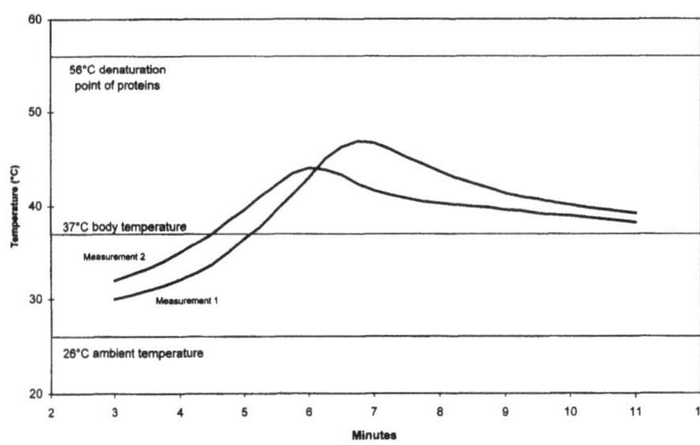

Fig. 1. Determination of temperature at the Palacos®–bone interface with normal blood circulation

Mechanical Testing

Mechanical tests were developed to investigate bending, impact, and fatigue behavior of bone cements. The results demonstrated that Palacos® offers strong mechanical stability, even after admixing the antibiotic gentamicin [3].

The Influence of Polymerization Heat on Bone Necrosis and Stem Loosening in Total Hip Replacement

Investigations of the influence of polymerization heat on bone necrosis and stem loosening in total hip replacement could verify that temperatures do not exceed 50 °C at the trochanter and 45.9 °C at the tip [4]. These temperatures are far below the denaturation point of proteins (56 °C). Several factors such as the presence of blood and moisture at the interface and the large surface area and poor heat conductivity of methylmethacrylate prevent the interface from experiencing the high rise in temperature that occurs at the center of the polymerizing cement mass [5] (Fig. 1).

Effects of Monomer Release from Bone Cements

After the heat problem was solved, the release of the monomer methylmethacrylate came under investigation [6]. It has been speculated that the release of monomer from bone cement was responsible for both aseptic loosening and the formation of pulmonary fat emboli. This speculation was based on the knowledge that the liquid monomer MMA is cytotoxic [8, 9]. Clinical investigations could show that blood levels of MMA are transiently elevated in patients undergoing arthroplasty using cement fixation (6 μg/ml 1 min after implantation) [10, 11]. Additionally, other factors such as loosening of a hip implant are known to raise levels again [11], even long after implantation. However, Wenda et al. [10] showed there was no correlation between the

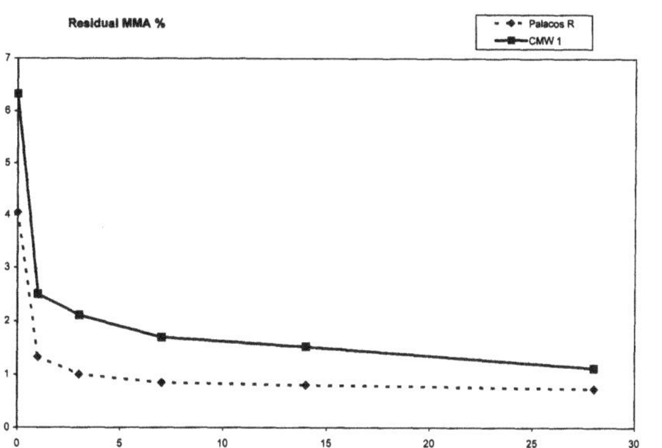

Fig. 2. Results for residual monomer versus implantation time

blood concentration of MMA and differences in the peripheral artery pressure (PAP) or respiratory rate (RR). Two hours after hardening of the cement, 3%–5% of residual monomer could be detected [6]. Our own investigations demonstrated that 10% of the monomer is released in decreasing amounts during the first 3 weeks, about 10% will stay in the bone cement for years, and 80% is consumed by continued polymerization [3, 12] (Fig. 2).

Wenzel et al. [14] could show that the released MMA can be metabolized in the Krebs cycle to CO_2 and water. In conclusion, no study could demonstrate that the monomer is responsible for loosening or formation of pulmonary fat emboli [15, 16]. But the level of monomer release should be kept as low as possible.

Fat and Bone Marrow Embolism

Weissman et al. [17] reported in the American volume of the *Journal of Bone and Joint Surgery* (JBJS) about intravenous methylmethacrylate after total hip replacement. The postoperative radiograph shows the filling of the vein by bone cement (Fig. 3).

With the increasing application of pressurization of the bone cement, the problem of intraoperative pulmonary embolization of air and medullary bone marrow increased. Ulrich et al. [18] showed that the pressure in the medullary canal during insertion of the cement and the stem can reach 5–6 bar and this high pressure is responsible for the circulatory problems, because bone marrow can be entrapped in the blood. They stated that a venting hole in the femur can prevent pressure from rising in the medullary space and therefore prevent embolization. They demonstrated this by transesophageal two-dimensional echocardiography. Emboli were shown in 8 of 12 patients without venting holes and only 2 of 12 with venting holes. These findings were confirmed in the British JBJS by Elmanraghy et al. [15].

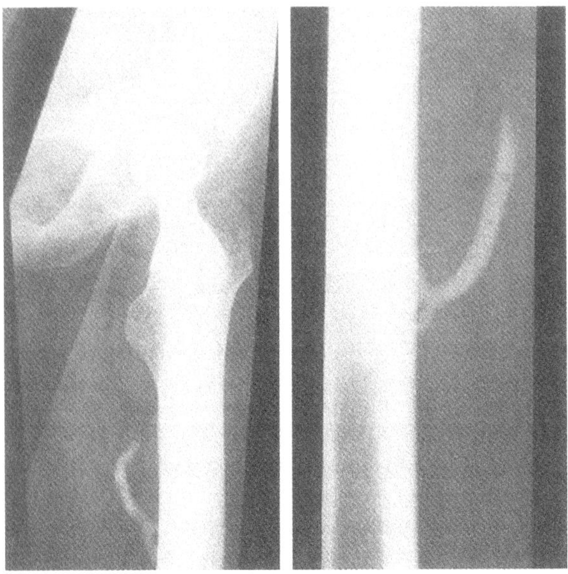

Fig. 3. Postoperative radiograph showing a serpiginous density extending into the soft tissues. The presence of a valve confirms the venous nature of this structure

The Meaning of Bone Cement Viscosity

The next problem that was heard from hospitals, especially in the United States, was that low viscosity bone cements penetrate spongy bone better than high viscosity bone cements.

A short time later, this assertion appeared in the British JBJS in a study by Benjamin et al. [19] on cementing technique and the effect of bleeding. They found that the bleeding pressure will force the bone cement out of the bone and blood can be entrapped in the cement. They showed that the bleeding pressure can vary from 6 cm to 36 cm of saline. In the experiments, they were able to vary the bleeding pressure (Figs. 4–7).

To overcome this problem, they concluded that the bone cement must be pressurized after injection for a better interlocking of the cement in the bone. The problem that could be caused by pressurizing low viscosity bone cements is shown in Figs. 6 and 7.

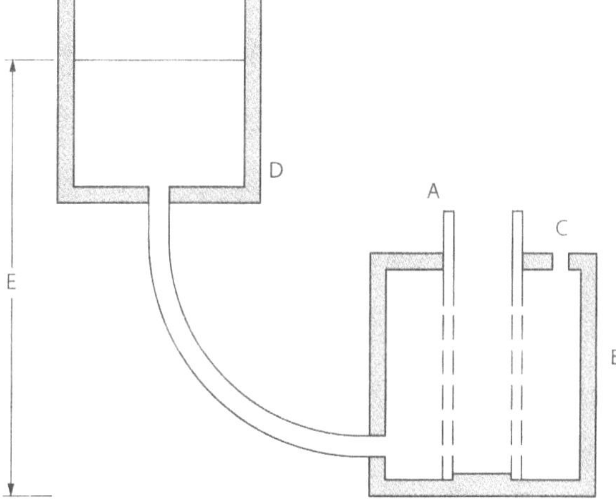

Fig. 4. Experimental apparatus. *A* fenestrated cylinder, *B* sealed chamber, *C* air vent, *D* blood reservoir, *E* measured height

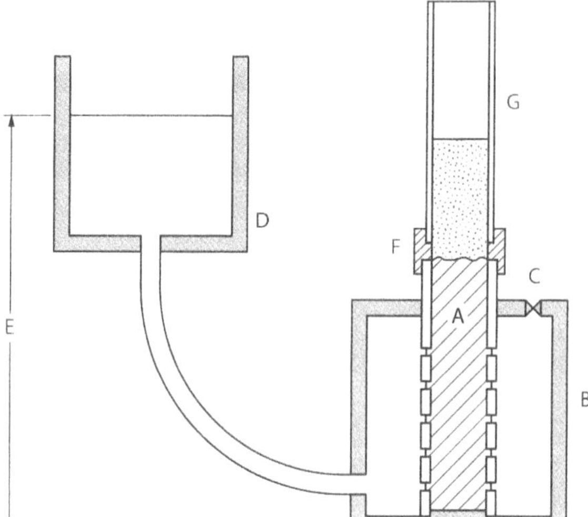

Fig. 5. Modified experimental apparatus. *A* fenestrated cylinder, *B* sealed chamber, *C* air vent, *D* blood reservoir, *E* measured height, *F* interconnection, *G* water reservoir

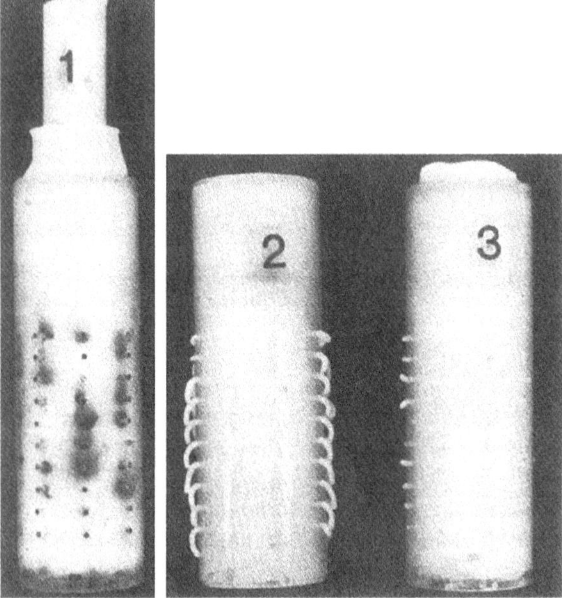

Fig. 6. The modified experiment. There was ingress of blood into the bone cement and consequent displacement of cement (specimen *1*). The different amounts of cement extruded are obvious at 2 min (specimen *2*) and 6 min (specimen *3*) after mixing

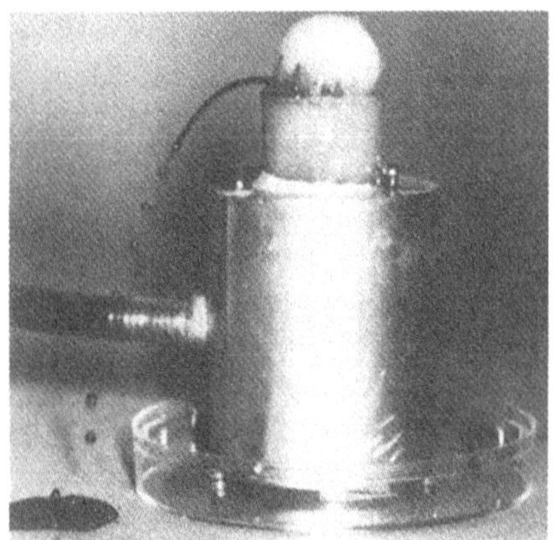

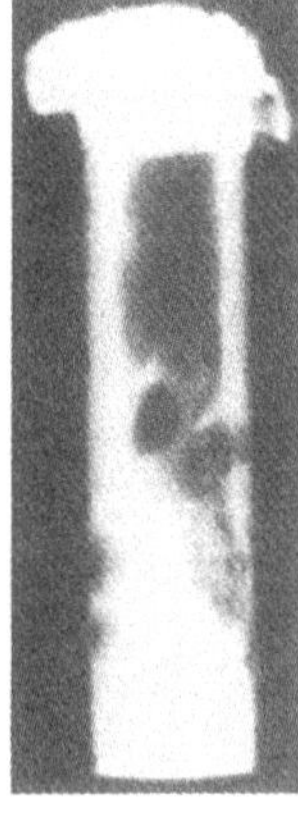

Fig. 7. During pressurization, blood is forced out at the top of the cylinder. The radiograph of a cement column shows large voids of blood

New Mixing Techniques

In the mid 1980s, vacuum mixing of bone cements to improve their mechanical properties was performed. As a high viscosity bone cement, Palacos® R could not be vacuum mixed at room temperature. Therefore, we started cooling the Palacos® R and found a temperature of about 4 °C to be best for vacuum mixing. New equipment came on the market and vacuum mixing increased. We found that cooling Palacos® R is not performed in all hospitals in the right manner, so we considered how to overcome this slight disadvantage. The goal was a bone cement at room temperature with the same behavior at the start as cooled Palacos® R. The mechanical properties should be the same or even better than those of Palacos® R. In a series of slight variations on Palacos® R, we tried to fulfill these parameters. The result of this research study is Palamed® [20].

Summary

- PMMA bone cement has proven clinical efficacy
- Palacos® R and Palamed® are safe products
- Palamed® is a more convenient form of Palacos® R

References

1. Charnley J (1960) Anchorage of the femoral head prosthesis of the shaft of the femur. J Bone Joint Surg Br 42:28–30
2. HW Buchholz (1969) Private correspondence to Kulzer
3. Kühn K-D (2000) Bone Cements. Springer, Berlin Heidelberg New York
4. Biehl G, Harms J, Hanser U (1974) Experimentelle Untersuchungen über die Wärmeentwicklung im Knochen bei der Polymerisation von Knochenzement. Arch Orthop Unf Chir 78:62–69
5. Reckling FW, Dillon WL (1977) The bone-cement interface temperature during total joint replacement. J Bone Joint Surg 59A:80–82
6. Rudigier J, Scheuermann H, Kotterbach B, Ritter G (1981) Restmonomerabnahme und -freisetzung aus Knochenzementen. Unfallchirurgie 7:132–137
7. Hollander L, Kennedy RM (1951) Dermatitis caused by autopolymerizing acrylic restoration material. Dent Dig 57:213
8. Endler F (1953) Die allgemeinen Materialeigenschaften der Methylmethacrylat-Endoprothesen für das Hüftgelenk und ihre Bedeutung für die Spätprognose einer Hüftarthroplastik. Arch Orthop Unf Chir 46:35
9. McLaughlin RE, Reger SI, Barkalow JA, Allen MS, Di Fazio CA (1978) Methylmethacrylate: a study of teratogenicity and fetal toxicity of the vapor in the mouse. J Bone Joint Surg 60A:355–358
10. Wenda K, Degreif J, Runkel M, Ritter G (1993) Pathogenesis and prophylaxis of circulatory reactions during total hip replacement. Arch Orthop Trauma Surg 112:260–265
11. Svartling N, Pfaffli P, Tarkkanen L (1986) Blood levels and half-life of methylmethacrylate after tourniquet release during knee arthroplasty. Arch Orthop Trauma Surg 105:36
12. Gil Albarova J, Lacleriga A, Barrios D, Canadell J (1992) Lymphocyte response to polymethylmethacrylate in loose total hip prostheses. J Bone Joint Surg 74:825
13. Scheuermann H, Ege W (1987) Aufbau und Zusammensetzung handelsüblicher Knochenzemente. In: Willert H-G, Buchhorn G (eds) Aktuelle Probleme in der Chirurgie und Orthopädie, Band 31. Knochenzement, pp 17–20

14. Wenzl H, Garbe A, Nowak H (1973) Experimentelle Untersuchungen zur Pharmako-kinetik von Monomethylmethacrylat. In: Erlacher PH, Zemann L, Spitzy KH (eds), pp 1–16
15. Elmaraghy A, Humeniuk B, Anderson GI, Schemitsch EH, Richards RR (1998) The role of methylmethacrylate monomer in the formulation and hemodynamic outcome of pulmonary fat emboli. J Bone Joint Surg Br 80B:156–161
16. Crout DMG, Corkill JA, James ML, Ling RSM (1979) Methylmethacrylate metabolism in man. Clin Orthop 141:90–95
17. Weissman BN, Sosman JL, Braunstein EM, Dadkhahipoor H, Kandarpa K, Thornhill TS, Lowell JD, Sledge CB (1984) Intravenous methyl methacrylate after total hip replacement, J Bone Joint Surg Am 66(3):443–450
18. Ulrich C, Burri B, Wörsdorfer O, Heinrich H (1986) Intraoperative transoesophageal two-dimensional echocardiography in total hip replacement. Arch Orthop Trauma Surg 105:274–278
19. Benjamin JB, Gie GA, Lee AJC, Ling RSM (1987) Cementing technique and the effect of bleeding. J Bone Joint Surg Br 69:620–624
20. Specht R, Kühn K-D (1998) Palamed and Palamed G: new bone cements. Abstracts. North Sea Biomaterials, The Hague, p 169

III Properties of Bone Cements

Handling Properties of Polymethylmetacrylate Bone Cements

K.-D. KÜHN

Introduction

According to the International Standards Organization (ISO) 5833 (1992), every manufacturer of bone cement is obliged to present a detailed and if possible graphic representation of the handling properties of the cement for the user. This is undoubtedly necessary as the nurse in the operating theatre mixes the two-component materials and thus produces the final product. For this purpose, we have worked out a method of testing the handling properties. On that basis, we have described the handling behaviour of all bone cements on the market. Moreover, we think it is important to show the influencing factors and their effects on the quality of the final product.

Materials and Methods

We tested 38 plain and 20 antibiotic-loaded bone cements.

Determination of the Working Properties

Mix an original package which has been maintained in an air-conditioned room (standard climate: 23±1 °C, 50±10% humidity, possibly also 18±1 °C or 25±1 °C) for at least 12 h according to the manufacturer's instructions in a porcelain crucible and start a stopwatch when the liquid is first added to the powder. After thorough mixing, determine the time at which the dough is homogeneous (Fig. 1; end of mixing phase = phase I).

Check every 5 s whether the dough still sticks to the finger (Fig. 1, waiting phase = phase II).

Working time starts when the dough is no longer sticky (Fig. 1, working phase = phase III).

Knead the dough until it can no longer be joined smoothly (end of the working phase), and the prosthesis can no longer be placed (Fig. 1, start of hardening phase = phase IV).

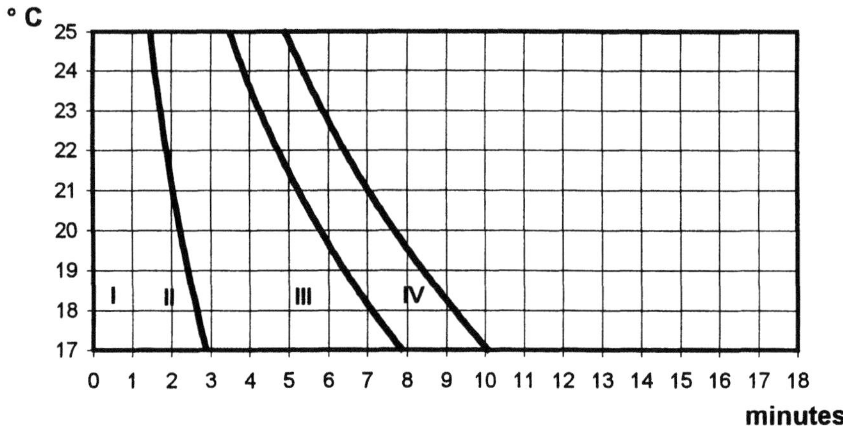

Fig. 1. Working curves of bone cement

The setting time is the time of complete hardening, which can be recognized by the hard sound of a cement ball hitting the table. All property and setting times are reported in minutes:seconds.

The examined cements are defined as low viscous, medium viscous, and high viscous, using the above-mentioned method. According to Kühn (2000), we define these properties as follows:

1. Low viscous (=low): Bone cements with a long-lasting liquid to low-viscous wetting phase. The material usually remains sticky for 3:00 min. In its working phase, the viscosity quickly increases and the dough becomes warm fast. The end of the working phase and the time of hardening are not more than 1:00–2:00 min apart.

2. Medium viscous (=medium): Bone cements with a low-viscous wetting phase. As a rule, the material is no longer sticky after 3:00 min at the latest. During the working phase, the viscosity remains more or less the same and increases slowly and continuously. In that phase the cement behaves like a high-viscous material. Hardening occurs 1:30–2:30 min after the end of the working phase.

3. High viscous (=high): Bone cements with only a short wetting phase which quickly lose their stickiness. During the working phase the viscosity remains unchanged and slowly increases towards the end of this phase. Generally, the working phase is especially long. Hardening occurs 1:30–2:00 min after the end of the working phase.

Results and Discussion

Mixing Phase

The cements differ greatly as early as the mixing phase. Some cements can easily be mixed, others can only be homogenized with great difficulty and utmost caution. Breusch et al. (1999) studied the state of the cementing technique in total hip arthroplasty in Germany using a questionnaire, and found that the mixing sequence according to the manufacturer's instructions is observed in only two-thirds of all cases. The mixing phase is by no means trivial. In this process, so many air bubbles are mixed into the dough by thorough mixing that the porosity of the material is high and mechanical stability endangered (Jasty et al. 1990). This phenomenon was described by Charnley (1970) when bone cements were first used: the more powerfully and longer the dough is mixed, the more porous it will be!

Many studies show the influence of porosity on the mechanical properties of bone cements (Lee et al. 1973, 1978; Kummer 1974; Haas et al. 1975; Debrunner 1976; Kusy 1978; Müller 1979; Miller and Krause 1981; Demarest et al. 1983; Jasty et al. 1984, 1991; Lautenschlager et al. 1984; Connelly et al. 1987; Linden 1988; Schreurs et al. 1988). Similar studies were carried out by De Wijn et al. (1972, 1975a, 1975b), which additionally, like Debrunner (1976), describe the mechanism of pore formation and the mechanical properties of porous and non-porous materials. Apparently the form of the mixing vessel and the spatula, as well as the speed of mixing and the number of strokes, also have an influence on the homogeneous result. Of immense importance – especially during manual mixing – is the observation that careful kneading when the dough is no longer sticky can subsequently significantly reduce porosity (Eyerer and Jin 1986).

Apart from the described cause for the inclusion of air, it must be taken into account that air bubbles are already included through the polymer powder and – especially by faulty use of vacuum-mixing systems – monomer bubbles can easily appear, which may develop during the evaporation of the monomer while evacuating the system or later during polymerization under high pressure (Oest et al. 1975). The formation of bubbles caused by the boiling monomer is one of the main problems when developing mixing systems under vacuum (Draenert 1988).

The influence of vacuum-mixing on the pores results in an improvement of the bending strength of Palacos® R by 15%–30% (Lidgren et al. 1984; Wang et al. 1993, 1994, 1995). Centrifugation is another way of achieving pore reduction (Burke et al. 1984; Rimnac et al. 1986). Davies et al. (1989), for example, found a reduction of porosity from 9.4% to 2.9% for Simplex® P, when centrifuged, resulting in an increase of fatigue strength.

Working Phase

The working phase is the time in which the surgeon can easily apply the cement into the femur. For manual application, the cement must no longer be sticky in this phase and the viscosity must not be too high. In this parameter, the cements differ significantly. So far, no one has succeeded in comparing all cements – probably because of the missing determination method – in order to characterize this phase, which is eminently important in practice.

Evidently, the working phase of the cements changes with the use of mixing systems, since with these the user need not wait until the cement is no longer sticky. However, a not-too-low viscosity in the early phase must be guaranteed. If this is not the case, the applied cement cannot withstand the bleeding pressure in the femur. Blood is included in the cement (Draenert 1988), and this inclusion must be looked upon as a distinct weak point with a high fracture risk (Soltesz et al. 1998a, b). This phenomenon is the main problem when using low-viscous cements since these are often applied to the body at much too early a point because of their short working phase (Draenert et al. 1999).

In the following section, we will describe the working phase of all examined bone cements because of their importance for surgeons. Only few bone cements examined show a working phase that is longer than 3 min. Some cements tested by our method have a long working phase, but the viscosity

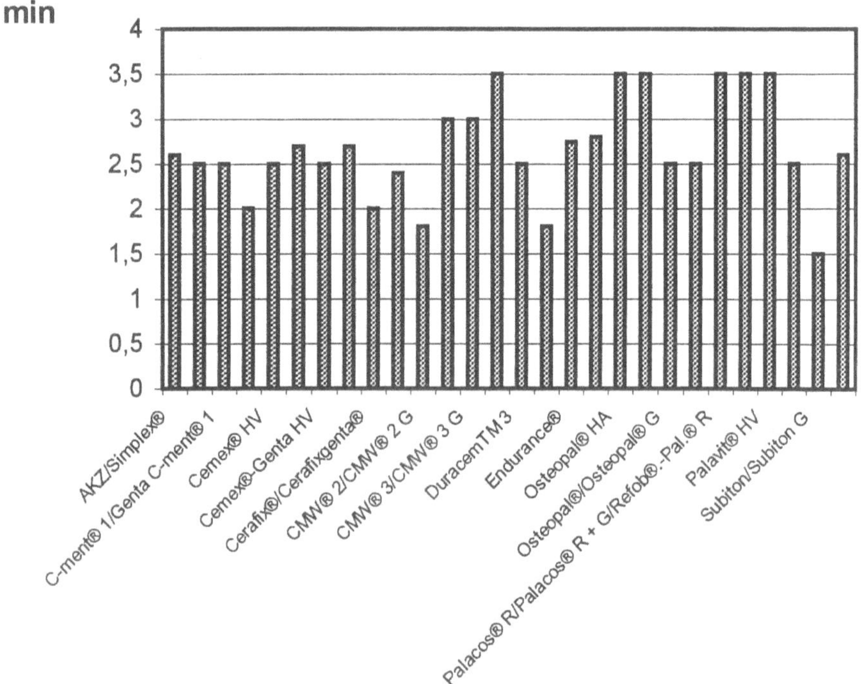

Fig. 2. Working times of all tested bone cements at 23 °C (room and components) according to Kühn (2000)

during that time will be so high that insertion of the dough and fixation of the prosthesis can not easily be performed.

Otherwise, some low-viscous cements show a relatively long working phase which is not usual for such material. Within the working time the viscosity varies significantly from low- to high-viscous dough and therefore the time for application is really short (Fig. 2).

Palacos® R, Palacos® with gentamicin, Refobacin®-Palacos® R, Osteopal® HA, Osteopal® VS, Copal, Palamed® and Palamed® G show a working phase longer than 3 min.

Krause et al. (1982) described in detail the viscosity of the most important cement types on the market at that time. CMW® 1 has the highest viscosity of all examined cements. Therefore, it is only suitable for manual mixing. Simplex® P is regarded as medium viscous, whereas Zimmer® LVC, AKZ, and Sulfix® 6 are characterized as low viscous. Wixson and Lautenschlager (1998) even regard Palacos® R as more viscous than CMW® 1. De Wijn et al. (1975a) claim that Palacos® R is twice as viscous as Simplex® P 5 min after the start of mixing but has only one-third of the viscosity of CMW® 1. Ferracane and Greener (1981) also reported on the viscosity of different bone cements.

Hardening Phase

The hardening phase indicates the moment from which the surgeon can expect the cement to be completely hardened. The manufacturer can only carry out in vitro tests of this phase and determine the hardening times in the laboratory under defined conditions (e.g. temperature, humidity). While often a complete package of cement is handled in the laboratory and thus a large quantity with a long-diameter cement ball is tested, the surgeon aims at a cement thickness of not more than 2–5 mm under operation conditions in vivo. The hardening behaviour under operation conditions – particularly under the influence of the temperature in the operating theatre, the temperature of the components, the body temperature, and the cement thickness – can significantly differ from the statements in the manufacturer's instructions. The many different factors influencing the polymerization kinetics of polymethylmetacrylate (PMMA) are probably the reason for this discrepancy.

According to Breusch et al. (1999), the moment at which the cement is applied to the femur and the acetabulum is standardized to a large extent (in about 88% of all cases), the mixing time of the bone cement, however, is standardized in only two-thirds of all cases. In slightly more than 50% of all cases, the cement is apparently still mixed by hand, and only in about 40% without pre-cooling of components and mixing vessels.

The pre-cooling of the monomer, the polymer, and the mixing vessels and the use of vacuum systems during mixing result in a significant reduction of the number and volume of pores. As a consequence, a considerable improvement of the fatigue strength of bone cements has been described (Demarest et al. 1983; Keller and Lautenschlager 1983; Wixson et al. 1985, 1987; Draenert 1988; Soltesz and Ege 1993; Soltesz et al. 1998a, b).

An essential prerequisite for the use of vacuum mixing systems, however, is their correct use. Nothing is worse than an incorrect mixing technique. In the Swedish Hip Arthroplasty Register, the vacuum mixing technique is recommended – but only with absolutely correct use (Malchau and Herberts 1998). The authors report on a learning effect in the users of mixing systems; this was reflected in the fact that satisfactory clinical results were achieved only after several years of experience.

An interesting discovery in the present study is the dependence of the determined times on the ambient temperature and the components; not every operating theatre is air-conditioned and has constant conditions during an operation.

Take note: Handling properties of bone cements are extremely dependent on temperature.

Low-Viscosity Bone Cements

All low-viscous bone cements being investigated have a liquid wetting phase at the beginning. Therefore, a homogeneous mix will be easily performed. A relatively long low-viscous phase follows and the nurse and surgeon have to wait for the end of the sticky phase. At the end of the working phase, the viscosity of low-viscous bone cements will rapidly increase, so that the time for insertion and fixation is usually short. Therefore, it is often observed when using low-viscous bone cements that the dough is inserted too early or too late. If the dough has been inserted too early, the viscosity of the material is too low to prevent the dough from intermixing very quickly with blood because of the higher blood pressure. This becomes apparent when the entire prosthesis together with the bone cement gets pushed out by the blood flowing back due to a hydraulic pressure (Benjamin et al. 1987). On the other hand, the optimal time of application can easily be missed because the material hardens quickly. In our opinion, these disadvantages mean that low-viscous bone cements may only be used if the staff is well trained in handling such material.

Table 1. Handling times of low-viscous bone cements at 23 °C (room and components)

Cements	End of sticky phase (min:s)	End of working phase (min:s)
Allofix® G	3:45	6:15
C-Ment® 3	4:00	6:00
Cemex® LV	3:00	6:00
Cerafix® LV	4:30	6:30
CMW® 3	4:00	7:00
Duracem™ 3	3:45	6:15
Endurance®	3:15	6:00
Osteobond®	4:15	7:00
Osteopal®	3:00	5:30
Palavit® LV	3:00	5:30
Zimmer® dough-type	4:00	6:40

To demonstrate the problem of short handling characteristics of low-viscous bone cements, we have summarized all our results in Table 1. To that purpose we have put together the end of the sticky phase and the end of the working phase of all low-viscosity bone cements that were examined at 23°C in this study.

Contrary to high- and medium-viscous cements, vacuum mixing (Demarest et al. 1983) of low-viscous bone cements may only be performed under a low vacuum of approximately 550 mbar. This vacuum will not be sufficient to fully eliminate the microporosity (Draenert 1988; Draenert et al. 1999). Vacuum mixing at room temperature at a pressure of 150 mbar resulted in boiling monomer due to its vapour pressure as a function of temperature. Chilling of low-viscous bone cement before mixing to reduce the viscosity which is well known for high-viscous bone cements is not valid because of the extremely late setting time.

For some low-viscous bone cements it is required to use the material only in mixing systems (Allofix® G, C-Ment® 3, Duracem 3, Genta C-Ment® 3, Palavit® LV). In our opinion this procedure may not reduce the disadvantages of the material. Nevertheless, using low-viscous bone cements only in mixing

Table 2. Factors influencing the properties of bone cements (Kühn 2000)

Relative humidity: <40%	Prolongation of working times for 1–3 min consider: OR – fully conditioned OR – partially conditioned winter: cold summer: warm
Storage in primary container	Water-uptake through PE/paper/Tyvek Change of mixing properties ⇒ Better: storage in aluminum pouch
Temperature of powder/liquid	at 23 °C: setting e.g. after 6–7 min (ISO) at 2–6 °C: setting e.g. after 12–14 min (ISO)
Pre-warmed mixing vessel	High temp.: faster setting Low temp.: delayed setting
Admixing of antibiotics	Inhomogeneous mixture
Mixing sequence	Strictly follows the package insert, else: uneven wetting of polymer ⇒ inhomogeneous mixture
Mixing parameters	Strictly follow the package insert, e.g. 20 ml liquid+40 g powder, or 30 ml+60 g or 5 ml+10 g, else: change of cement properties
Effects of resterilization – Heat	 Destruction of benzoyl peroxide ⇒ no curing
– Irradiation	Fission of polymer chain, reduction of molecular weight ⇒ totally different material properties
– Gas resterilization	High ethylene oxide residues can only be done using a validated ventilation program

OR, operating room

systems might easily mask the present problems because of missing the direct contact to the material. Therefore the risk of a false application may increase. Besides having detailed knowledge about the material properties, the user has to also be well trained in the mixing devices. Malchau and Herberts (1998) explained the unsatisfactory clinical results of bone cements applied by inexperienced staff using the vacuum-mixing system and the mixing device. The authors observed that with increasing experience the clinical results will lead to better overall results.

Because of the importance of the handling behaviour of bone cements for the user, this property has to be adjusted from batch to batch by the manufacturer as indicated. Therefore, it is important to know which factors can influence the handling properties of the cements (Table 2). If, for instance, the polymer component is stored at a relative humidity of less than 40%, the working time is prolonged. It is of importance whether the operating theatre is fully or partly conditioned.

In conformance with the manufacturers' instructions, no package should be used unless it is in its original state and there are no doubts of its tightness.

Because of the high dependence of the polymerization of the temperature, not only the temperature of the room but also of the components and mixing devices has to be taken into account. Principally cooler ambience or components result in slower polymerization and lower viscosity, while on the other hand, higher temperatures have the opposite effect.

Mixing vessels may quickly warm up by handling in the operating room (OR) before the mixing. Draenert et al. (1999) describe how long it takes for the pre-cooled powder to reach the appropriate temperature.

Setting times may vary dramatically with different room temperatures, mixing vessels, or components. Meyer et al. (1973) showed the dependence of time for Simplex® P. At an ambient temperature of $4\,^{\circ}C$ they found a setting time of 60 min, while at $37\,^{\circ}C$ the material had already hardened after 3 min.

Additives admixed to the supplied cement components are very critical. In industry, production follows strict legal requirements to assure a constant quality. With a later manual blending of additives there is a great risk of getting an inhomogeneous dough. In addition, the quality of the mechanical properties drops significantly, especially when adding substances to the liquid (Lautenschlager et al. 1976).

The mixing sequence should be followed as to the manufacturer's suggestions, otherwise inhomogeneities may be the consequence (Draenert et al. 1999). The wetting phase is normally tested and optimized by the manufacturer thus giving best mixing results.

One should also refrain from changing the powder/liquid mixing ratio in order to influence the viscosity. Otherwise, the cement properties and possibly mechanical strength may be spoiled.

Resterilization of cement components is strictly forbidden, as all methods have different influences on the material. Heat, for example, degrades the initiator benzoyl peroxide (BPO) thus preventing polymerization. Resterilization by irradiation of originally gas-sterilized powders changes the cement properties by degradation of the polymer chains. When resterilizing using ethylene oxide (EO), one has to consider that not all EO sterilization methods can be used and that there is a high EO absorption in the powder. The gas has to be desorbed using a valid venting procedure.

References

Benjamin JB, Gie GA, Lee AJ, Ling RS, Volz RG (1987) Cementing technique and the effect of bleeding. J Bone Joint Surg Br 69:620–624

Breusch SJ, Draenert K, Draenert Y, Boerner M, Pitto RP(1999) Die anatomische Basis des zementierten Femurstieles. Z Orthop 137:101–107

Burke DW, Gates EI, Harris WH (1984) Centrifugation as a method of improving tensile and fatigue properties of acrylic bone cement. J Bone Joint Surg 66:1265–1273

Charnley J (1970) Acrylic cement in orthopaedic surgery. Williams and Wilkins, Baltimore

Connelly TJ, Lautenschlager EP, Wixson RL (1987) The role of porosity in shrinkage of acrylic cements. Transactions of the 13th Meeting of Society 12:114

Davies JP, Jasty M, O'Connor DO, Burke DW, Harrigan TP, Harris WH (1989) The effect of centrifuging bone cement. J Bone Joint Surg 71B:39–42

Debrunner HU (1976) Untersuchungen zur Porosität von Knochenzementen. Arch Orthop Unfall-Chir 86:261–278

Demarest VA, Lautenschlager EP, Wixson RL (1983) Vacuum mixing of methylmethacrylate bone cement. Trans Soc Biomat 6:37

Draenert K (1988) Zur Praxis der Zementverankerung. Forschung und Fortbildung in der Chir. des Bewegungsapp. 2, München: Art and Science

Draenert K, Draenert Y, Garde U, Ulrich C (1999) Manual of cementing technique. Springer, Heidelberg

Eyerer P, Jin R (1986) Title Influence of mixing technique on some properties of PMMA bone cement. J Biomed Mat Res 20:1057–1094

Ferracane JL, Greener EH (1981) Rheology of acrylic bone cements. Biomat Med Dev Artif Organs, 9:213–224

Haas SS, Brauer GM, Dickson GA (1975) Characterization of polymethyl-methacrylate bone cement. J Bone Joint Surg (Am) 57 A:380–391

(ISO) International Standards Organization 5833 (1992)

Jasty M, Jensen NF, Harris WE (1984) Porosity measurements in centrifuged and uncentrifuged commercial bone cement preparations. Poster present: 2nd World Congress of Biomaterials, Washington

Jasty M, Davies JP, O'Connor DO, Burke DW, Harrigan TP, Harris WH (1990) Porosity of various preparations of acrylic bone cements, Clin Orthop Rel Res 259:122–129

Jasty M, Maloney WJ, Bragdon CR, O'Connor DO, Zalenski, EB, Harris WH (1991) The initiation of failure of cemented femoral components of hip arthroplasties. J Bone Joint Surg 73B:551–558

Keller JC, Lautenschlager EP (1983) Experimental attempts to reduce acrylic porosity. Biomat Med Dev Art Org 11:221–236

Krause WR, Miller J, Ng P (1982) The viscosity of acrylic bone cements. J Biomed Mater Res 16:219–243

Kühn K-D (2000) Bone Cements. Springer, Berlin Heidelberg New York

Kummer FJ (1974) Bone cements: effects of pressurization on structure and mechanical properties. Trans Orthop Res Soc 21:245–149

Kusy RP (1978) Characterization of self-curing acrylic bone cement. J Biomed Mater Res 12:271–305

Lautenschlager EP, Jacobs JJ, Marshall GW, Meyer PR Jr (1976) Mechanical properties of bone cements containing large doses of antibiotic powders. J Biomed Mat Res 10:929–938

Lautenschlager EP, Strupp SI, Keller JC (1984) Structure and properties of acrylic bone cement. In: Duchaynep Hasting GW (ed) Functional behavior of orthopedic biomaterials, vol II. Applications, CRC Series in structure-property relationships of biomaterials. Boca Raton FL: CRC Press

Lee AJ, Wrighton JD (1973) Some properties of polymethylmetacrylate with reference to its use in orthopedic surgery. Clin Orthop 95:281

Lee AJ, Ling RS, Vangal SS (1978) Some clinically relevant variables affecting the mechanical behaviour of bone cement. Arch Orthop Traumat Surg 92:1–18

Lidgren L, Drar H, Moller J (1984) Strength of polymethylmethacrylate increased by vacuum mixing. Acta Orthop Scand 55:36–541

Linden U (1988) Porosity in manually mixed bone cement. Clin Orthop 231:110–112

Malchau H, Herberts P (1998) Prognosis of Total Hip Replacement. Scientific Exhibition. Presented at the 65th Annual Meeting of the American Academy of Orthopedic Surgeons, New Orleans, USA

Meyer PR Jr, Lautenschlager EP, Moore BK (1973) On the setting properties of acrylic bone cement. J Bone Joint Surg 55A:139–156

Miller J, Krause WR (1981) The effect of viscosity on intrusion and handling of bone cement. Orthop Trans 5:352–353

Müller K (1979) A practice orientated study of the complex "Processing and handling – Application-Resultant Properties of autopolymerizing PMMA bone cements". Werkstofftech 10:30–36

Oest L, Müller K, Hupfauer K (1975) Die Knochenzemente. Ferdinand Enke Verlag Stuttgart

Rimnac CM, Wright TM, McGill DL (1986) The effect of centrifugation on the fracture properties of acrylic bone cements. J Bone Joint Surg 68A:281–287

Schreurs BW, Spierings PT, Huiskes R, Slooff TJ (1988) Effect of preparation techniques on the porosity of acrylic cements. Acta Orthop Scand 59:403–409

Soltész U Ege W (1993) Influence of mixing conditions on the fatigue behaviour of an acrylic bone cements. 10. Europ Conf of Biomaterials, Davos, pp 138

Soltész U, Schäfer R, Kühn K-D (1998a) Effect of vacuum mixing on the fatigue behaviour of particle containing bone cements. Abstracts: North Sea Biomaterials, The Hague, pp 69

Soltész U, Schäfer R, Kühn K-D (1998b) Einfluß von Anmischbedingungen und Beimengungen auf das Ermüdungsverhalten von Knochenzementen. 1. Tagung des DVM-Arbeitskreises „Biowerkstoffe", 89–94

Wang JS, Franzèn H, Toksvig-Larsen, T (1994) A comparison of seven bone cement mixing systems. Acta Orthop Scand 65(260):62

Wang J-S, Franzèn H, Jonsson E, Lidgren L (1993) Porosity of bone cement reduced by mixing and collecting under vacuum. Acta Orthop Scand 64:143–146

Wang J-S, Franzèn H, Toksvig-Larsen S, Lidgren L (1995) Does vacuum mixing of bone cement affect heat generation? Analyses of four cement brands. J Appl Biomater 6:105–108

de Wijn JR, Sloof TJ, Driessens FC (1972) Characterization of bone cements. Arch Orthop Unfall-Chir 72:174–184

de Wijn JR, Driessens FC, Slooff TJ (1975a) Dimensional behavior of curing bone cement masses. J Biomed Mat Res 9:99–103

de Wijn JR, Slooff TJ, Driessens FC (1975b) Characterization of bone cements. Acta Orthop Scand 46:38–51

Wixson RL, Lautenschlager EP (1998) 9. Methyl Methacrylate. In: Ed Callaghan JJ, Rosenberg AG, Rubash HE (eds) The adult hip. Lippincott-Raven, Philadelphia, pp 135–157

Wixson RL, Lautenschlager EP, Novak M (1985) Vacuum mixing of methylmethacrylate bone cement. 31st Annual Orthop Res Soc (ORS) Meeting in Las Vegas

Wixson RL, Lautenschlager EP, Novak MA (1987) Vacuum mixing of acrylic bone cement. J Arthroplasty 1:141–149

Mechanical Properties of Bone Cements

K.-D. KÜHN, R. SPECHT, W. EGE, H.-J. KOCK

Introduction

Poly(methyl methacrylate) (PMMA) bone cements fill the space between the prosthesis and the bone; this connection is only a mechanical bond. The irregularities of the surface of the bone and the penetration of the cement into these irregularities are of great importance for the bond. The PMMA-layer has the effect of an elastic buffer between the prosthesis and the bone. Thus, the main function of the bone cement is to transfer load from the prosthesis to the bone or increase the load-carrying capacity of the surgical construct. Due to its low rigidity it can reduce the stress concentrations at the interface of the bone. The PMMA-cement must endure considerable stresses when used for in vivo applications. Thus, strength characteristics are important for its clinical success. If the imposed stresses are higher than the load-carrying capacity of the cement, then a cement fracture may occur leading to the failure of the construct. Therefore, it is evident that accurate and extensive data on the mechanical properties of a particular cement being used are indispensable for its optimum use in surgery. The effectiveness of surgical bone cement must be viewed in the light of its mechanical properties. Generally, there are two possibilities for the determination of the mechanical strength of bone cements: static tests and dynamic tests.

Static mechanical properties are those derived from tests conducted at a low rate of loading such as tensile, compressive, flexural (bending), impact or shear strength. These tests can be carried out at different times after hardening, or the specimens can be stored in water or Ringer's solution at different degrees. The rigidity of the cements can be determined from the tensile, compressive or bending tests as modulus of elasticity.

In the standard for bone cements ISO 5833 (1992) 'Implants for surgery – Acrylic resin cements' the following quasi-static mechanical tests are described (Figs. 1, 2).

Additionally, the cements can be tested dynamically, that is, in a long-term load alternation test. Such tests have not yet been included in the present ISO 5833. However, for the revised version being written at present, there are three different proposals for a dynamic fatigue test.

Such tests can be carried out as a tensile, compressive or bending test. Usually the fatigue properties are determined in a bending test, as the neces-

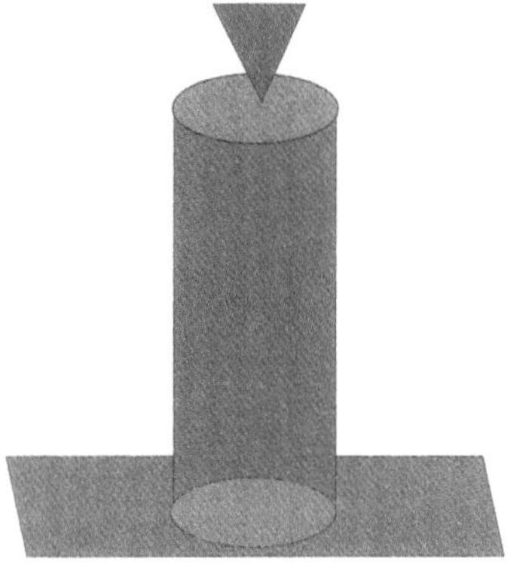

Fig. 1. Method of determination of the compressive strength – ISO 5833 (1992)

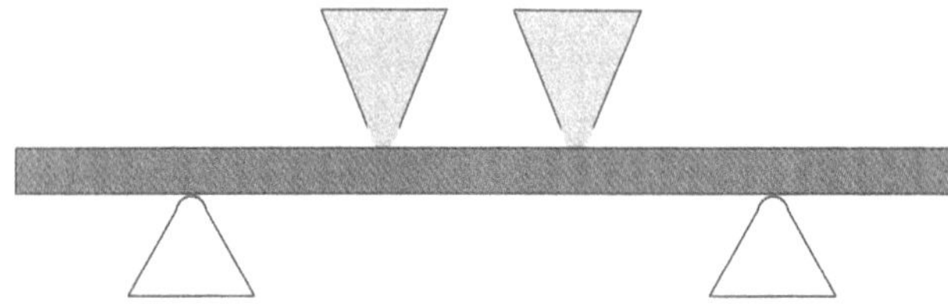

Fig. 2. Method of determination of the bending modulus and bending strength – ISO 5833 (1992)

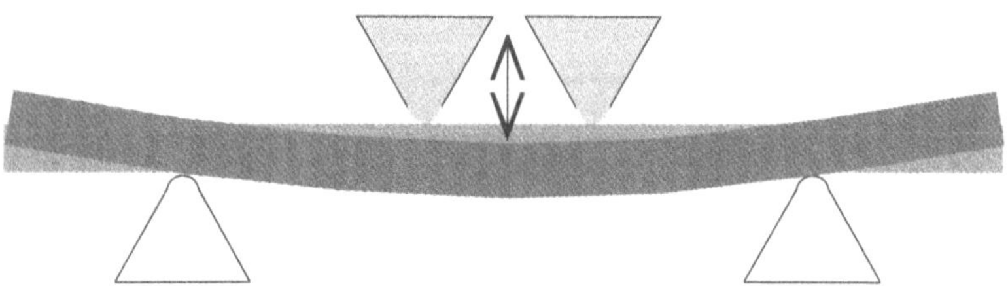

Fig. 3. Long-term load cycling test (fatigue) – Soltesz (1994)

sary devices are more simple. However, such tests are extremely time consuming, as the number must be at least 10^7, and the number of load alternations per second should not exceed 10, and preferably be between 3 and 5. Soltesz (1994) modified the bending test of ISO 5833 to a dynamic fatigue test. For that test the specimens are saturated with water for about 4 weeks at 37 °C and the tests run in Ringer's solution at 37 °C. The method of Soltesz (Fig. 3) is one of the three proposals discussed for the revision of the ISO 5833.

Ege et al. (1998a) pointed out the differences between conventionally and vacuum-mixed specimens of a commercial bone cement. Whereas the quasi-static values of the bone cements on the market do not differ significantly it is obvious that the materials are weakened with increasing cycle number. In

which case the differences between the PMMA-bone cements on the market
are extremely high.

Results and Discussion

Firstly, the results of several static tests conducted by different investigators
are reported after the implementation of the ASTM as well as ISO standard
for PMMA-bone cements. Ungethüm and Hinterberger (1978) reported the
first comparative results of several static tests, mainly the compressive
strength according to ISO 5833/1 (1979) and the impact strength of 5 different bone cements. Lee et al. (1978) pointed out that bone cements have sufficient strength as early as 2 h after polymerization, which will slightly increase during the slow post-curing, but will by then have almost attained the
upper limit. Lautenschlager et al. (1976) showed that the addition of aqueous
solutions of antibiotics has even more disastrous consequences for the mechanical strength of bone cements. In 1981 Edwards and Thomasz tested 8
different bone cements. Further comparative studies of various bone cements
have frequently been published. However, they frequently only dealt with a
few cement types and some questions of particular interest. Hansen and
Jensen (1992) compared 10 different bone cements strictly according to ISO
5833. Comparative studies of various bone cements have frequently been
published; however, they often concern only a few types of cement and particular questions on cement properties. New cements especially are readily introduced in comparative studies with the so-called old pharmaceutical specialties Simplex® P or Palacos® R. Kindt-Larsen et al., (1995) for example
compared Boneloc®, a newly developed bone cement, with 4 other bone cements registered for the United States. Meanwhile, Boneloc® had to be with-
drawn from the market (Havelin et al. 1995). Usually only some of the cement's properties are compared in these studies, and the methods used cannot always be applied to all cements (Ege 1993). Ege (1994) reported results
of static tests on 10 different bone cements. He determined bending strength
and impact strength according to DIN 53435 (Dynstat method), modulus of
elasticity in the bending test according to DIN 13907, a standard for dental
materials. This unsatisfactory situation results in continuing consumer uncertainty, as they cannot easily compare the cements on the market. Recently,
Lewis (1997) published another detailed review on the cement properties of 6
cements, mainly versions for the United States market.

Meanwhile bone cements have been for sale for over 30 years and today 38
different materials are available (22 PMMA-cements without antibiotics and
16 with antibiotics), but many studies still make a comparison impossible
because several different standards for metals or plastics are used. Moreover,
some cements are hard to obtain.

As mentioned, today the most relevant quasi-static mechanical tests are
described in ISO Standard 5833 (1992) in detail (compressive strength, bending strength, bending modulus). Therefore, an overview and comparison of
all bone cements available on the market, examining that standard in partic-

ular will be demonstrated as well as new fatigue results of some important bone cements according to Soltesz' method. Additionally, the glass transition temperature of all bone cements on the market has been determined.

ISO Compressive Strength – Results

We found cements that have compressive strengths of above 100 MPa and others that do not reach much more than the lower limit of 70 MPa.

Palavit®LV, Osteobond®, C-ment® 3, Palavit® HV, Endurance®, Durus® H, CMW® 1, CMW® 2, CMW® 3, Cerafix® and Cemex® HV belong to the first group. Many of these are low viscous (Fig. 4). The high values of Palavit® cements can be explained with their special cross-linking ingredient ethylene glycole dimethacrylate. This yields in a polymer matrix that is more rigid when exposed to compressive influence. The material is more brittle then with a high modulus and may break more easily under stress. Thus, a high compressive strength together with a high modulus of elasticity seems to be disadvantageous in surgery regarding the aimed function of the cement as an elastically buffering interface. An upper limit for the compressive strength should be demanded in the standard.

Compressive strengths above 100 MPa are also reported for Sulfix® 6 in the literature (Edwards and Thomasz 1981). Similar data for other low viscous cements are reported by Hansen and Jensen (1992), e.g. for CMW® 3: 100–104 MPa. Krause et al. (1980), however, found only 73 MPa for Zimmer®

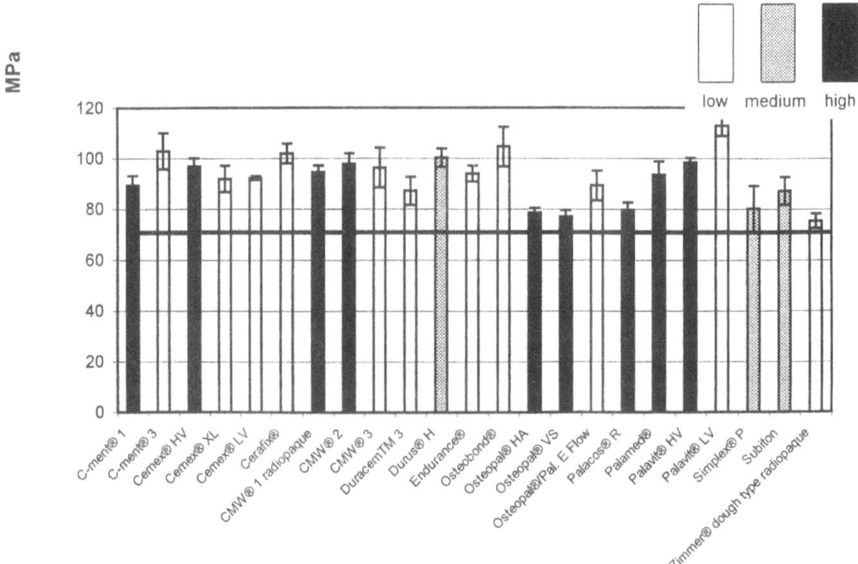

Fig. 4. Compressive strength of plain bone cements – ISO 5833 (1992)

dough-and Bargar et al. (1983) 81 MPa for the same cement, in spite of its low viscosity.

Some manufacturers advertise the high compressive strengths of their products. The distributor's results for Cerafix®, for instance, 107 MPa, correspond well with the data found by us. For Cemex® cements compressive strengths above 120 MPa and modulus far beyond 3000 MPa are claimed. That should result in considerable brittleness. We could not detect these high values.

In the second group Osteopal® HA, Osteopal® VS, Palacos® R, Simplex® P and Zimmer® dough-type are found. The low compressive strengths of Osteopal® VS and Osteopal® HA may well be explained by their high content of filler.

Our results correspond with those of Hansen and Jensen (1992) and Kindt-Larsen et al. (1995), who found compressive strengths of high viscosity more or less below 90 MPa. Different results are given especially for Simplex P. While we found an average of about 80 MPa, Kindt-Larsen et al. (1995) found almost 100 MPa, independent of the mixing technique. Edwards and Thomas (1981) come to the same results. The high compressive strengths of low viscous cements compared to high viscous variants are confirmed by our study.

Besides the preparation of the test specimens and their storage the test parameters are of decisive importance. Lee et al. (1978) had already pointed that out earlier. We only want to cite the importance of the "strain rate" here, leading to results between 80 and 122 MPa. This holds also true for the modulus (Lee et al. 1978).

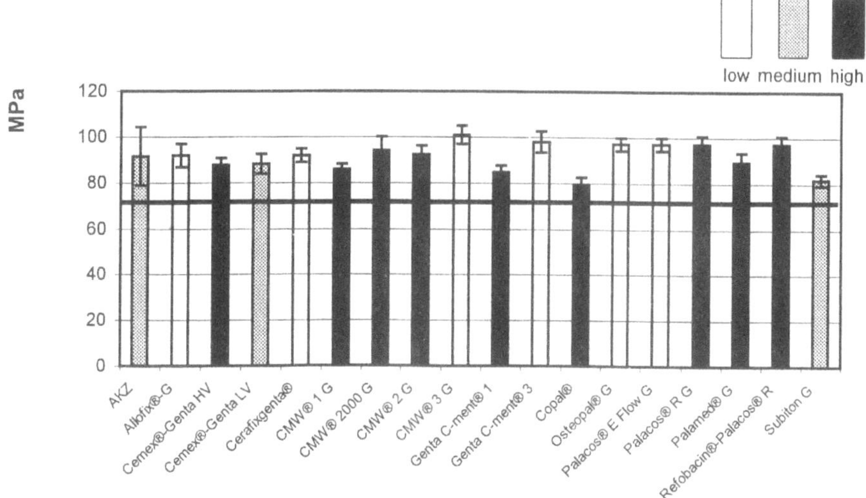

Fig. 5. Compressive strength of antibiotic bone cements – ISO 5833 (1992)

The results of antibiotic-loaded cements are generally a little below those of the plain materials. The antibiotics are never an integrated part of the polymer matrix, thus weakening the cement, though the percentage of the added antibiotic is low (Fig. 5).

However, there seem to be exceptions. For some antibiotic bone cements the compressive strength is higher than for the plain versions (all Palacos® products, Cerafixgenta®, CWM® 3G). This was also observed by Ungethüm and Hinterberger (1978), who found a higher compressive strength for Refobacin®-Palacos® R than for Palacos® R.

Lee et al. (1978), on the other hand, found a significant decrease of the compressive strength with the increase of added antibiotic. Edwards and Thomasz (1981) come to similar results for Palacos®R with (89 MPa) and without (100 MPa) antibiotic.

ISO Bending Strength – Results

Test specimens defined by the relevant standard are used. They have to be stored for 50 h in water or Ringer's solution at 37 °C. Because of the water storage another factor has to be taken into account: the ability of water absorption depending on the kind of copolymers used.

The low strength of the Cemex® products and the values of all Subiton® samples below the limit of the standard are noticeable.

From the literature the low bending strength of Zimmer® cements is known (48 MPa, Hansen and Jensen 1992) as well as 56 MPa (Weber and

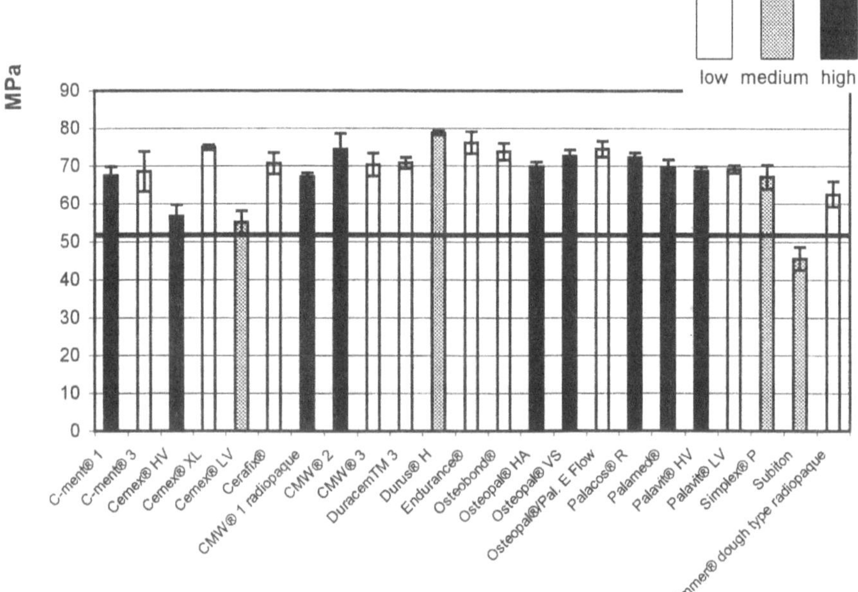

Fig. 6. Bending strength of plain bone cements – ISO 5833 (1992)

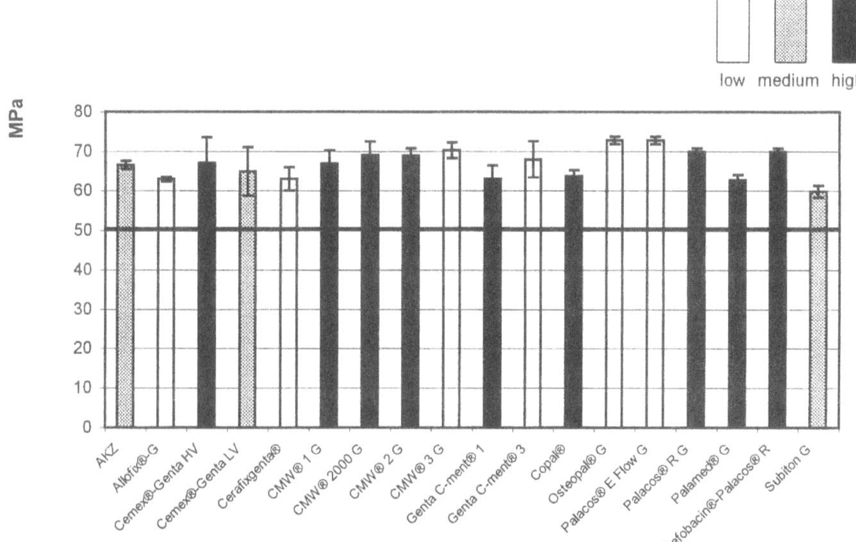

Fig. 7. Bending strength of antibiotic bone cements – ISO 5833 (1992)

Bargar 1983). All other cements show more or less 70 MPa (Fig. 6). Different from Hansen and Jensen (1992), who report the highest result for Simplex® P (74 MPa), we always found low values. Moreover, CMW® cements and Palacos® R show higher strength in our study compared to Hansen and Jensen (1992).

The low strength of the Cemex® products and the values of all Subiton® samples below the limit of the standard are noticeable. All these results are quite similar for the antibiotic cements (Fig. 7). Noticeable are the high standard deviations for the Cemex® cements and CMW® 1G and CMW® 2000G.

ISO Bending Modulus – Results

The modulus of elasticity is known to be a measure for the stiffness of a material. It tells how much a material is deformed by stress (Fig. 8), the higher the modulus the less the material is deformed. The stiffness depends on the amount of absorbed water. Thus, the ISO 5833 requires a defined way and period of storage before testing. Lee et al. (1978) describe other influences.

All modulus found in our study, except for Subiton, fulfill the requirements of the standard. Yet all values were clearly above the lower limit of 1700 MPa (ISO 5833) (Fig. 9).

Different from its plain version Subiton G is above the lower limit here. The modulus of Copal® is comparatively lower, which might be explained with the high content of antibiotics.

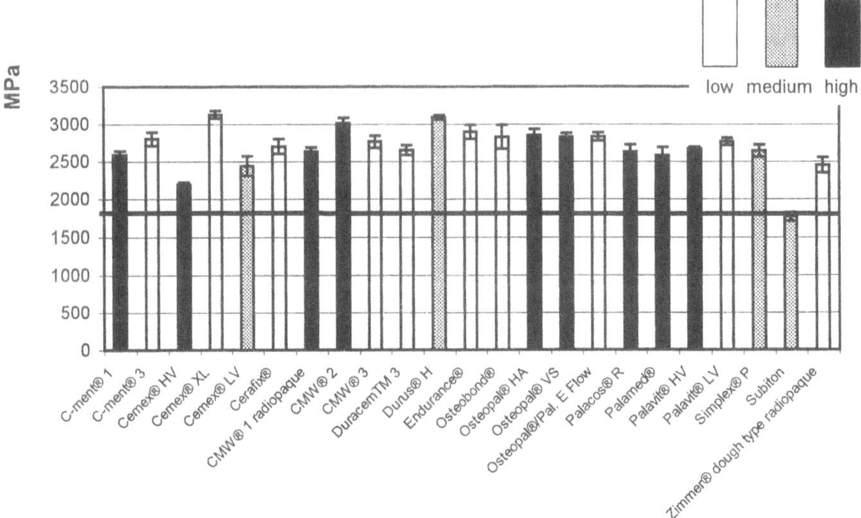

Fig. 8. Bending modulus of plain bone cements – ISO 5833 (1992)

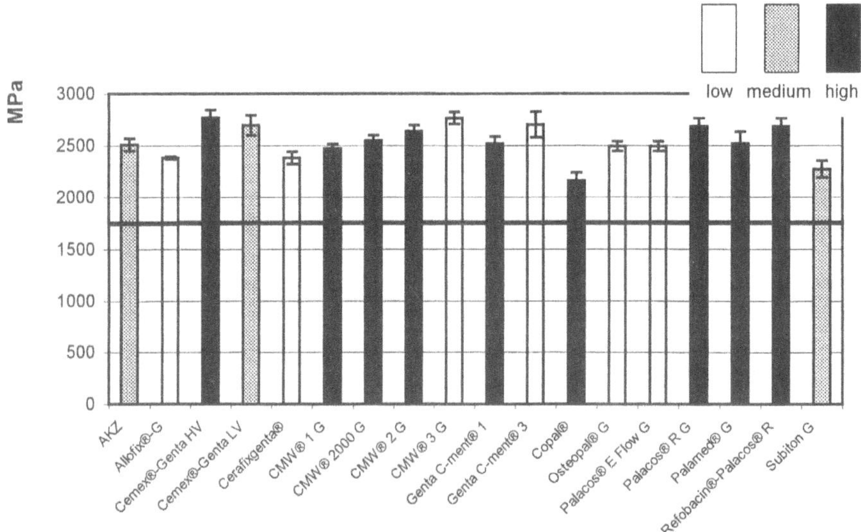

Fig. 9. Bending modulus of antibiotic bone cements – ISO 5833 (1992)

Table 1. Comparison of the 4-point bending strength and modulus: storage 16 h dry at 37 °C and 50 h wet at 37 °C (Kühn and Ege 1999)

Material	Batch	4-point modulus 16 h dry (MPa)	4-point modulus 50 h wet (MPa)	4-point bending strength 16 h dry (MPa)	4-point bending strength 50 h wet (MPa)
AKZ	820287 E	2789	2361	67.2	63.0
Refobacin®-Palacos® R	9022	3044	2681	68.7	62.9
CMW® 1G	Y070A40	2967	2379	64.3	61.6
CMW® 3G	Y069B40	3275	2624	69.1	62.7
Osteopal® G	9015	3077	2625	68.9	62.9
Copal®	0007	3087	2290	66.5	58.6

Table 2. Comparison of the bending modulus and the bending strength of ISO test specimens being stored for 16 h dry at 37 °C and 50 h wet at 37 °C, respectively (Kühn and Ege 1999)

Material	Batch	4-point modulus 16 h dry (MPa)	4-point modulus 50 h wet (MPa)	4-point bending strength 16 h dry (MPa)	4-point bending strength 50 h wet (MPa)
Simplex® P	148DD/822DD	2915	2665	51.7	50.5
Palacos® R	8909	3075	2697	71.7	68.3
CMW® 1	XO79R40	2964	2682	68.2	70.8
CMW® 3	YOO9L40	3275	2875	73.7	72.8
Osteopal®	9035	3049	2795	77.1	73.6

In our opinion, in general the water storage capacity (50 h) of ISO 5833 does not make sense. The results for dry- and water-stored samples do not differ sufficiently significantly to justify this time-consuming preparation. The specimens should either be stored in water until saturation (3–4 weeks) before testing or they should simply be tested dry.

Using the ISO method those cements have an advantage in that they have a slow water uptake. The differences in water absorption, though small, really seem to have an influence on the ISO bending strength.

Our results shown in Table 1 (antibiotic-loaded cements) demonstrate clearly water-storage results in lower mechanical strength. These results are only available after 2 days. By using dry specimens tested after 16 h the results are available the next day. Moreover, the effect of the different water uptake within the 2 days makes us think that this method is better for practice.

The examined plain bone cements showed similar results as described above. The bending strength, however, did not show significant differences when tested at 16 h dry and 50 h water-stored at 37 °C (Table 2).

Interesting in Table 2 are the extreme deviations for Simplex® P. While the regular test resulted in a bending strength of about 70 MPa, the samples

Table 3. Factors influencing the mechanical strength

	Decrease in mechanical strength	Increase in mechanical strength
Water uptake	↑	↓
Continuing polymerization	↓	↑
Release of monomer	↓	↑

tested in a different manner only produced 50.5 MPa. The following scheme holds true for a couple of mechanical tests of bone cements (Table 3).

After implantation of the cement dough into the femur and curing there are two subsequent effects: the continuing polymerization, normally resulting in a better mechanical strength, and absorption of water. This has a plasticizing effect and decreases the strength. Together with the absorption of water the release of residual monomer starts. A slow monomer release can result in worse mechanical strength, while a rapid diffusion should have a good influence on the mechanical strength (Kühn and Ege 1999).

Long-Term Load Cycling Test (Fatigue) – Results

For this study we compared cements with comparable initial viscosity to minimize the influence of differing mixability. It is known, for example, that low viscous cements are much less problematic as to the pores in the dough than are high viscous cements. One premise, of course, is the correct and steady way of mixing. We prepared all our test specimens by using the same mixing vessels and spatulas. Mixing was done according to the manufacturer's instructions by the same person. The materials used are listed in Table 4.

Table 4. Bone cements for fatigue testing

Cement (conventionally mixed)	Viscosity during mixing	Quasi-static starting point (MPa)	After 10^7 cycles	% of quasi-static values
Palacos® R	High	67.6	17.8	26.3
CMW® 1	High	57.1	12.3	21.5
Refobacin®-Palacos® R	High	60.4	17.0	28.0
CMW® 1G	High	61.5	14.1	23.0
Palamed®	Medium	62.0	17.6	28.0
Simplex® P	Medium	60.1	14.2	23.7
Palamed® G	Medium	58.6	17.4	30.0
AKZ	Medium	61.0	11.5	18.9
Osteopal®	Low	65.6	26.0	40.0
CMW®3	Low	59.7	10.4	17.3
Osteopal® G	Low	58.6	20.0	34.0
CMW® 3G	Low	60.0	6.2	10.4

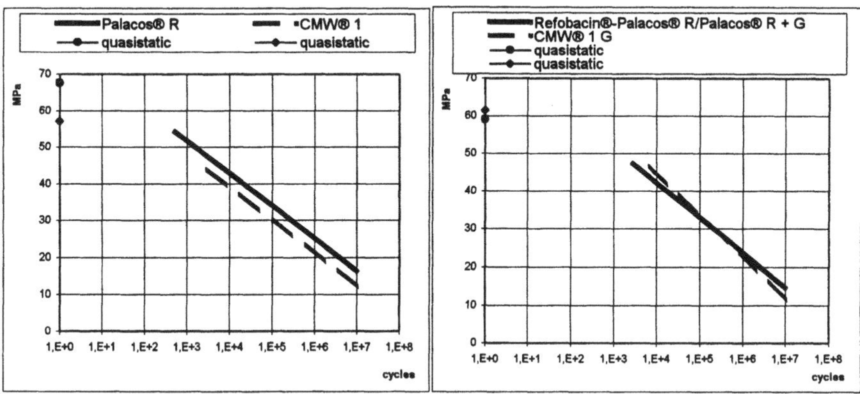

Fig. 10. Wöhler curves of high viscous bone cements (with and without antibiotic): Palacos® R and CMW®1

Comparing the most important high viscous cements CMW® 1 and Palacos® R, one can see that the quasi-static values differ a bit. For Palacos® they are higher than for all samples of CMW®1, which could already be stated in the tests according to ISO 5833, although this is not really significant. But CMW® 1 samples, with and without antibiotic, show a much lower fatigue strength than Palacos® R with and without antibiotic. Palacos® R with antibiotic is much better than plain CMW® 1. The differences given as percentage of the quasi-static values show that clearly (Fig. 10).

Maybe the difference can be explained by the content of gentamicin being twice as high in CMW® 1G (1.0 g base/40 g) as in Refobacin®-Palacos® R/Palacos® R with gentamicin (0.5 g base/40 g). That counts especially because the plain variant of CMW® 1 is weaker than Palacos® R. Different from Refobacin®-Palacos® R and Palacos® R with gentamicin the antibiotic variant of CMW® 1 starts at a higher level but then breaks down faster.

For the next comparison we used two bone cements (Palamed® and Palamed® G), which are principally regarded as highly viscous. Because of their significantly lower viscosity at the time of mixing, however, they are regarded and compared in this chapter as 'medium viscous'.

For the medium viscous cements we noted similar results. The quasi-static data were comparable here as well. Simplex® P and AKZ, however, showed a significantly lower fatigue strength compared to Palamed® and Palamed® G, respectively (Fig. 11).

It is an interesting observation for the 2 medium viscous cements that the fatigue strengths of the plain products are almost identical to those containing antibiotic. They both have a low initial viscosity allowing a low degree of pores to be reached. In the following medium viscous working phase the cements seem to behave similarly, though the working phase is clearly longer for Palamed® than for Simplex® P. Maybe this kind of viscosity behavior, together with the chemical composition, is the reason for the different results in fatigue testing.

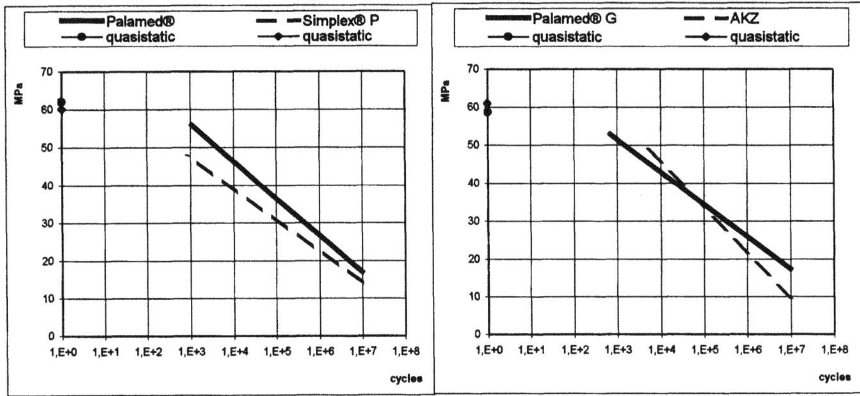

Fig. 11. Wöhler curves of medium viscous bone cements (with and without antibiotic): Palamed® and Simplex® P

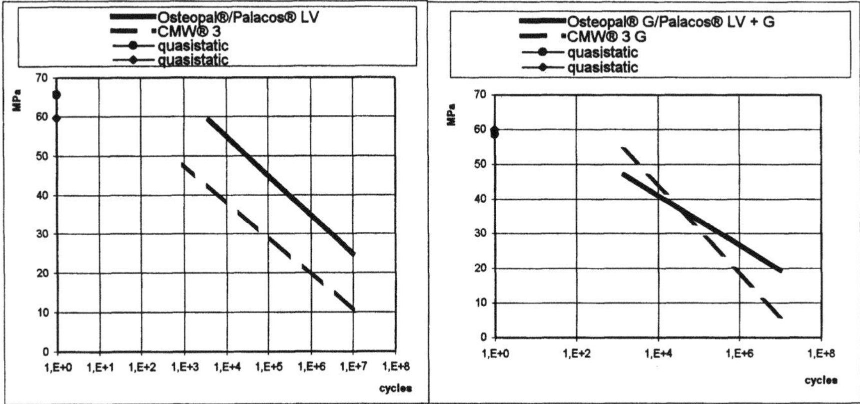

Fig. 12. Wöhler curves of low viscous bone cements (with and without antibiotic): Osteopal®/Palacos® LV/E Flow and CMW® 3

Another interesting factor is the influence of styrene copolymer Simplex® P and AKZ. It seems as if their water-uptake is slower and the specimens not yet water-saturated after the minimum storage time of 4 weeks in water at 37 °C. This would mean that the fatigue strength would be even worse testing the material after complete saturation with water.

The differences are especially significant for the low viscous cements (Fig. 12). Plain CMW® 3 already shows worse fatigue strength compared to Osteopal®. For the antibiotic variants CMW® 3G and Osteopal® G the differences are even higher. Similar to the high viscous types the high initial level of CMW® 3 can then drop dramatically. Lewis (1999) also describes very good fatigue behavior for Osteopal® mixed manually and under vacuum. The hand-mixed Osteopal® shows clearly better fatigue properties than the vacuum-mixed Simplex® P.

Glass Transition Temperature (According to Ege et al. 1998b)

Upon heating resins their state changes from glass-like and brittle to elastic. This physical law also applies to poly(methyl methacrylates), which also means to bone cements. Due to the distribution of the molecular weight, an exact transition temperature does not exist, only a softening range (Vieweg and Esser 1975).

In order to determine the glass transition temperature the specialist can use several methods: torsional fatigue testing, shear modulus determination and the dilatometric method (DSC). The DSC method is most frequently used and does not show significant differences between dry and water-saturated materials. The reason for this phenomenon seems to be that only small quantities of granulated material are used, which already dry up during the heating time (1 °C/min) (Ege et al. 1998b). The method we use gives results that can be reproduced in every respect, since we use a relatively large amount of material.

Specimens of the dimension $3 \times 3 \times 20$ mm were prepared; one half was stored dry at 37 °C and Tg determined after 24 h. The second half was stored at 37 °C in water and Tg was determined after 4 and 8 weeks using a dilatometer that exactly records the expansion of length in the case of increasing of temperature (1 °C/min) in the form of a graph.

When glass transition temperature (Tg) is attained, Brown's molecular micro movements are excited, which themselves are the reason for some changes in the material parameters. They influence the thermal expansion coefficient, the bending modulus and mechanical and electric absorption. The Tg depends on molecular weight, water content and, of course, on the molecular structure of the monomer used.

In the last few years, Tg has been used for additional characterization of bone cements (Thanner et al. 1995). Some researchers postulated that particularly the Tg of older pharmaceutical specialties was much too high, the materials were brittle and therefore often one of the reasons for loosening of the components.

New developments were started where the Tg can be adjusted to about 50 °C by using methacrylates with a longer alkyl side chain. Unfortunately, either only theoretical calculations on the composition had been made in these considerations or the few measurements were carried out on dry specimens.

The researchers dreadfully neglected the fact that bone cements always remain in a humid environment at 37 °C in the body after implantation and become saturated with water after only a few weeks. A plasticizing effect develops and Tg inevitably decreases (Ege et al. 1998b).

Basically the experiments show that the glass transition temperature clearly decreases by about 20 °C after water absorption (Fig. 13). Whereas there is no change in temperature when the samples are stored in a dry environment, a continuous decrease in temperature can be observed when stored in water at 37 °C. However, when the samples are water-saturated, there are no more changes.

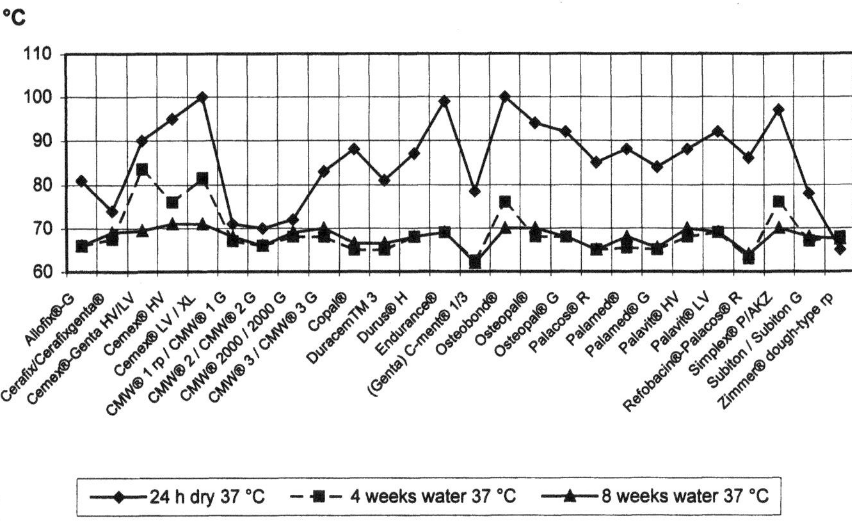

Fig. 13. Glass transition temperature

Here we can once again see that the glass transition temperature is directly proportional to the water absorbing properties of the different examined materials. Because of the comparatively high hydrophobic properties of styrene copolymers the examined samples of Cemex® cements, Osteobond® and Simplex® P after 24 h of storage have glass transition temperatures, which at first are relatively high and that are in contrast to all other materials still comparatively high (about 75 °C) after 4 weeks of storage in water. Obviously the water absorption of these bone cements with styrene copolymers is so slow that the glass transition temperature adapts itself correspondingly slowly to the temperatures of other cements. These, however, after 4 weeks of storage in water show nearly the same glass transition temperatures as samples that were stored in water for 8 weeks. For the styrene-containing cements CMW® 2000G as well as Endurance® this could not be observed.

The reason could be that both cements contain distinctly less styrene than Cemex®, Osteobond® and Simplex® P. According to this there were no significant changes after 4 weeks of storage. This observation could also be of great importance in determining the fatigue behavior according to Soltesz et al. (1998), since in these experiments it is assumed that the samples are water-saturated after storage in water at 37 °C for about 4 weeks.

Acknowledgements. I would like to thank Dr. Tuchscherer (Heraeus Kulzer GmbH & Co. KG) for the mechanical tests, Mrs. Maurer (Heraeus Kulzer GmbH & Co. KG) for the determination of glass transition temperatures, Dr. Soltesz and Dr. Schäfer (Fraunhofer Institute, Freiburg) for the fatigue tests Mrs. P. Kühn for translation and Mr. Krause (Merck Biomaterial GmbH) for the supply of the different cements.

References

Bargar WL, Heiple KG, Weber S, Brown SA, Brown RH, Kotzar G (1983) Contrast bone cement. J Orthop Res 1:92–120

Edwards RO, Thomas FGV (1981) Evaluation of acrylic bone cements and their performance standards. J Biomat Mat Res 15:543–551

Ege W (1993) Knochenzement. In: Planck H (ed) Kunststoffe und Elastomere in der Medizin. Kohlhammer GmbH, Stuttgart, pp 112–121

Ege W (1994) Material properties of PMMA bone cements. In: Buchhorn GH, Willert H-G (eds) Technical principles, design and safety of joint implants. Hogrefe & Huber Verlag, Göttingen, pp 49–53

Ege W, Kühn K-D, Maurer H. Tuchscherer, Chr (1998a) Physical and chemical properties of bone cements. In: GHIM Walenkamp (ed) Biomaterials in surgery. Thieme-Verlag, Stuttgart, pp 39–42

Ege W, Kühn K-D, Maurer H, Tuchscherer Chr (1998b) Glass transition temperature of various bone cements. North Sea Biomaterials Abstract Volume, The Hague, 177

Hansen D, Jensen JS (1992) Mixing does not improve mechanical properties of all bone cements. Manual and centrifugation-vacuum mixing compared of 10 cement brands. Acta Orthop Scand 63:13–18

Havelin LI, Espehaug B, Vollset SE, Engesaeter LB (1995) Early aseptic loosening of uncemented femoral component in primary total hip replacement: a series based on the Norwegian Arthroplasty Register. J Bone Joint Surg 77B:11–71

ISO (1979) International standard 5833/1. Implants for surgery-acrylic resin cements. Orthopaedic Application

ISO (1992) International standard 5833/2. Implants for surgery-acrylic resin cements. Orthopaedic Application

Kindt-Larsen T, Smith DB, Jensen JS (1995) Innovations in acrylic bone cement and application equipment. J Appl Biomat 6:75–83

Krause W, Krug W, Miller J (1980) Cement bone interface effect of cement technique and surface preparation. Orth Transactions 4:204

Kühn K-D, Ege W (1999) Influence of a change of storage conditions in ISO 5833 on the mechanical results. North Sea Biomaterials, Bordeau-Archacon

Lautenschlager EP, Jacobs JJ, Marshall GW, Meyer Jr., PR (1976) Mechanical properties of bone cements containing large doses of antibiotic powders. J Biomed Mater Res 10:929–938

Lee AJC, Ling RS, Vangal SS (1978) Some clinically relevant variables affecting the mechanical behaviour of bone cement. Arch Orthop Trauma Surg 92:1–18

Lewis G (1997) Properties of acrylic bone cements: state-of-the-art-review. J Biomed Mater Res (Appl Biomater) 38:155–182

Lewis G (1999) Relative influence of molecular weight and mixing method on the fatigue performance of acrylic bone cement: Simplex®P versus Osteopal®. In: Bone cement: practice and progress. Kings College Hospital, London

Soltész U (1994) The influence of loading conditions on the lifetimes in fatigue testing of bone cements. J Mater Sci Mater Med 5:654–656

Soltész U, Schäfer R, Kühn K-D (1998) Einfluß von Anmischbedingungen und Beimengungen auf das Ermüdungsverhalten von Knochenzementen. 1. Tagung des DVM-Arbeitskreises "Biowerkstoffe"

Thanner J, Freij-Larsson C, Karrholm J, Malchan H, Wesslen B (1995) Evaluation of Boneloc chemical and mechanical properties. Acta Orthop Scand 66:207–214

Ungethüm M, Hinternberger J (1978) Die Normung von Implantatwerkstoffen am Beispiel Knochenzemente. Z Orthop 116:303–311

Vieweg R, Esser F (1975) Polymethylmethacrylate. C. Hauser Verlag, München

Weber SC, Bargar WL (1983) A comparison of the mechanical properties of Simplex, Zimmer, and Zimmer low viscosity bone cement. Biomater Med Devices Artif Org 11:3–12

Mechanical Testing of Palamed®

R. SPECHT, K.-D. KÜHN, W. EGE, H.-J. KOCK

Introduction

Since the beginning of the 1960s, bone cement as we know it today has been widely used for a variety of indications, of which the most important is the fixation of endoprostheses in the hip, knee, and other joints. During that time, much experience with this material was gathered. Very importantly, it has been found that not only the properties of the cement itself are responsible for clinical success, but also the technique used for mixing and application. These findings led to modern cementation techniques, in which the use of systems for vacuum mixing and application is recommended [1].

Bone cements can be classified into groups with high or with low viscosity. In clinical practice, the former show better results than the latter [1–3]. The reason for this effect is seen today in the higher risk of mishandling when using low-viscosity cements. High viscosities were originally developed for earlier techniques in which the cement was mixed in open bowls and applied by hand. For this type of application, high viscosity was found to be optimal. But with modern cementing techniques, the use of mixing systems and mixing under vacuum conditions is recommended. Mixing in a vacuum reduces the porosity of the cement, thus improving its mechanical properties. With many of the available mixing systems, however, the results with high-viscosity cements are not optimal concerning porosity. It has been found that prechilling the cement before mixing reduces viscosity, thus improving the mixing results. As a result of prechilling, however, the setting time of the cements is prolonged by several minutes. With respect to operation time, this has to be seen as a clear disadvantage.

The goal in the development of Palamed® and Palamed® G bone cements was to decrease viscosity early on for easier and more effective mixing in mixing systems without going so far as to result in a low viscosity cement. The properties important for convenient use and good clinical results were to resemble those of the well-known and proven Palacos® R cement as closely as possible.

Composition

Looking at its composition, it would seem very simple to produce a bone cement. In reality, bone cement is a very complex system in which all components must work together like toothed gears. Any change in composition has an influence on the properties of the cement. When developing a bone cement, these mutual influences have to be taken into account. In the past, a number of publications presented only single aspects of the improvements of various new compositions. Other aspects seem to have been forgotten and the cements did not show the expected results in clinical practice.

To achieve the desired results, the same ingredients as those in the well-known existing product were used for the new cement. The slightly reduced viscosity of Palamed® is the result of only small changes in composition, and no new substances were used. The amount of the radiopacifying agent ZrO_2 was reduced. The reason for this is the improved quality of modern x-ray machines, and the smaller amount of ZrO_2 is sufficient to produce excellent x-ray images. In addition, recent experiments indicate that the type of radiopacifier could have an influence on osteolysis in the region of the implant. These results, however, must be clearly elaborated.

As a result of slight modifications in composition, the viscosity of Palamed® is reduced in the first mixing phase. It has to be mentioned that Palamed® is nevertheless far from being a low-viscosity cement.

Handling

The effect of the reduced viscosity can be clearly seen by comparing porosity.

Experiments were performed by mixing Refobacin®-Palacos® R prechilled to 4 °C and Palamed® G stored at 22 °C, defined as room temperature in various mixing systems. The overall porosity was measured by ascertaining the density of the cured cements (P. Spierings, unpublished data). The results are presented in Table 1.

In each group of cement, the best results (i.e., the lowest porosity) were achieved using the Optivac® system. On the other hand, the porosity of samples produced from Palamed® G is lower than with Refobacin®-Palacos® R,

Table 1. Comparison of overall porosity of Palamed® G mixed at 22 °C and Rebofacin®-Palacos® R prechilled to 4 °C. All levels are given in percent

Mixing method	Palamed® G	Refobacin®-Palacos® R
Hand-mixed	6.9±1.0	7.7±0.8
Optivac	0.3±0.2	0.7±0.6
Cemvac	0.8±0.2	1.3±0.5
Summit bowl	1.8±0.7	4.0±1.2
Summit syringe	1.8±0.9	2.8±1.3

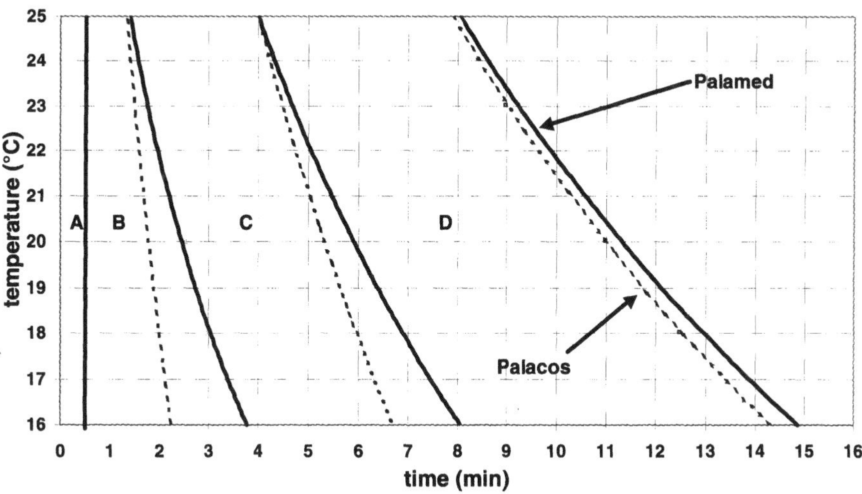

Fig. 1. Comparison of the handling properties of Palamed® and Palacos® R. *A* mixing phase, *B* waiting phase, *C* working phase, *D* setting phase

even if the Palamed® G is not prechilled but used at normal room temperature. The setting time of Palamed® G is also shorter than that of prechilled Refobacin®-Palacos® R. The results clearly show that the slight reduction in viscosity results in improved handling.

One consequence of the reduced viscosity is that the so-called doughing time, where the cement still sticks to the gloves, is slightly longer, so that surgeons using the cement by hand must wait a little longer than with Refobacin®-Palacos® R.

The time/temperature diagrams for both cements are compared in Fig. 1.

Mechanical Properties

Judging from frequency, the most important indication for bone cement is fixation of endoprostheses, e.g., in the hip or knee. In these cases, the mechanical requirements on cement are high. The international 5833 ISO standard [4] defines minimum values for the mechanical properties of bone cements as well as the methods for measuring those properties. According to this standard, compressive strength, bending strength, and the bending modulus are to be tested.

The mechanical properties of Palamed® G were evaluated according to this standard. In Fig. 2, the results are compared with those of Refobacin®-Palacos® R measured in the same way. The dotted lines in all figures indicate the minimum values defined by the ISO 5833. In all the three points mentioned above, no significant differences between Palamed® G and Refobacin®-Palacos® R can be detected. As for bending strength, one can see the well-known effect of the admixture of an antibiotic reducing mechanical strength.

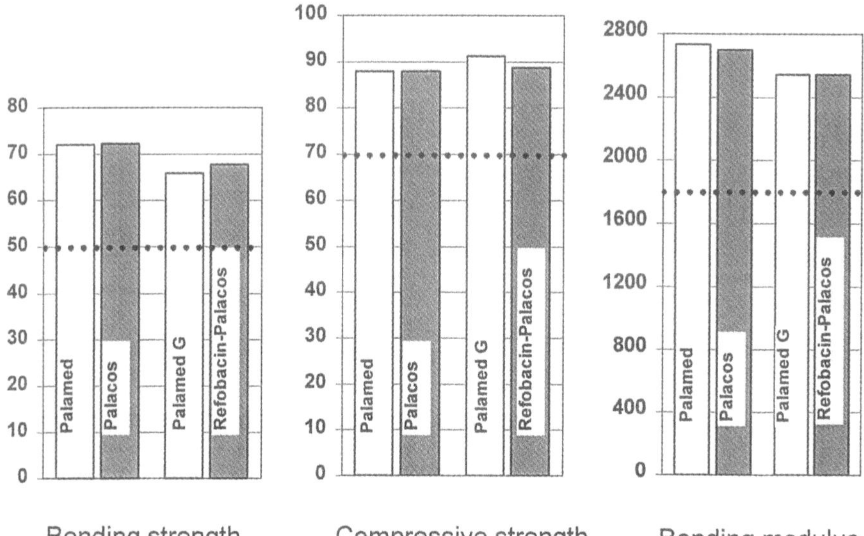

Fig. 2. Mechanical properties of Palamed® vs. Palacos® and Palamed® G vs. Refobacin®-Palacos® R according to ISO 5833 norms. All data are given in MPa. *Dotted line* indicates ISO 5833 requirements

Fatigue

The above methods are used for measuring the so-called static strength of bone cements. But because patients move and walk, the dynamic properties have to be tested as well. These measurements are shown in the description of fatigue behavior. All materials show decreasing strength with increasing numbers of cycles. Whereas for metals a stress limit normally exists below which the material will last forever, such a limit does not exist for polymers.

Although test conditions for static strength are standardized in the ISO 5833, no standard exists at present for fatigue testing. For this testing, we chose a method very close to that for bending strength as described in the ISO 5833. Sample size and geometry were identical to those required for ISO 5833, and the samples were saturated in Ringer's solution. Measurement was performed at 37 °C in Ringer's solution in load-controlled four-point bending by applying sinusoidal loads at a frequency of 5 Hz. The method follows Wöhler's procedure, in which samples are stressed with a defined load until fracture (U. Soltesz, unpublished data).

The results of our tests are listed in Fig. 3. As for static values, no differences were seen between the two plain or the two antibiotic-loaded cements. The reduction in mechanical strength by the addition of antibiotics, known for a long time, can be seen as well.

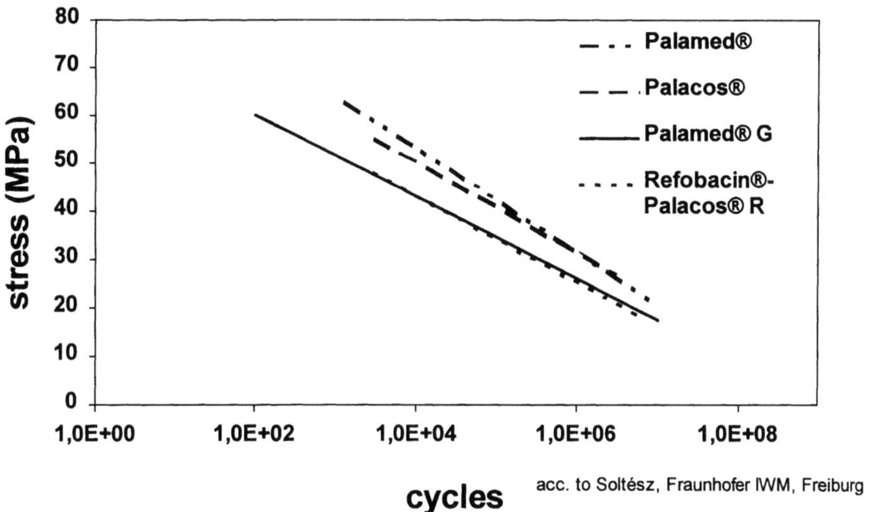

Fig. 3. Fatigue testing of Palamed® and Palacos® R, with and without gentamicin, mixed in a vacuum according to Soltész, Fraunhofer IWM, Freiburg, Germany

Release of Gentamicin

Antibiotics are added to bone cements in order to prevent infection from the implant. The special problem during implantation is that many germs have a high affinity to artificial surfaces. Once adhered, germs may be covered by a bioslime which protects them from natural metabolism and attack by antibiotics. In addition, fibrous tissue cells are prevented from adhering, thus preventing tissue integration of the implant. Gristina [5] described this effect as a "race for the surface". The solution to these problems is the admixture of antibiotics to the cement, resulting in high local concentrations of antibiotics in the implant surroundings immediately after implantation so that germs are prevented from adhering, thus reducing the risk of infection. The effectiveness of this method was proven in the Norwegian Hip Register [2, 6]. As one result of this study, it was clearly shown that the combination of local delivery of antibiotics from the bone cement in combination with systemic antibiotic treatment definitely reduced the infection rate. These results are also confirmed by the Swedish Hip Register [1], where antibiotic-loaded Palacos® R was found to be the best cement.

The release of gentamicin from bone cement is part of the quality control for each batch of bone cements from Biomet Merck (Darmstadt, Germany). The testing is performed according to standardized and validated procedures. Defined samples of the cement are produced and leached in buffer solution at 37 °C. After 24 h, the solution is changed. Measurement of the concentration of eluted gentamicin is performed according to the diffusion test described in the 1997 Pharmacopoea Europaea.

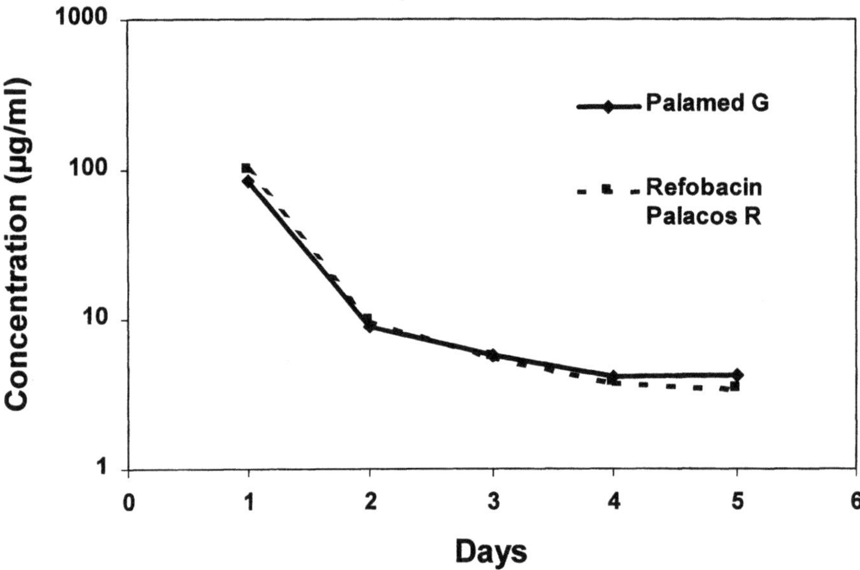

Fig. 4. In vitro release of gentamicin from Palamed® G and Refobacin-Palacos® R

The results of the experiments clearly show that in vitro Palamed® G and Refobacin®-Palacos® R have the same excellent release characteristics: very high levels during the first day followed by protracted release for the following days. It is known from clinical trials that in vivo and in vitro studies show the same antibiotic release behavior. For this reason, it can be concluded that Palamed® G will show in vivo the same release characteristics as Refobacin®-Palacos® R.

Summary

Palamed® and Palamed® G are not actually new products but represent further developments of well-known and proven bone cements. With slight modifications in composition, the excellent properties of the existing cements, including their mechanical parameters, could be retained, whereas the slight reduction of viscosity in the beginning of the mixing phase created an optimal bone cement for use with modern vacuum cementing techniques.

References

1. Malchau H, Herberts P (1998) Prognosis of total hip replacement. Scientific exhibition presented at the 65th annual meeting of the American Academy of Orthopedic Surgeons. New Orleans, USA
2. Havelin LI, Espehaug B, Lie SA Engesæter LB, Furnes O, Vollset SE (2000) Prospective studies of hip prostheses and cements. Scientific exhibition presented at the 67th annual meeting of the American Academy of Orthopedic Surgeons. Orlando, USA
3. Havelin LI et al (1995) The effect of the type of cement on early revision of Charnley total hip prostheses. J Bone Joint Surg Am 77A:1543–1550
4. International standard ISO 5833 (1992) Implants for surgery – acrylic resin cements. First edn. pp 11–15
5. Gristina AG (1994) Implant failure and the immuno-incompetent fibro-inflammatory zone. Clin Orthop 298:106–118
6. Espehaug B et al (1997) Antibiotic prophylaxis in total hip arthroplasty. J Bone Joint Surg Br 79B:590–595

IV Cementing Technique

Cementing Technique in Total Hip Replacement: Factors Influencing Survival of Femoral Components

STEFFEN J. BREUSCH

Abstract. This article gives an overview of the current status of modern cementing techniques for femoral component anchorage. The rationale of cemented hip arthroplasty and factors influencing long-term outcome are discussed. The aim during cement application is to establish a durable interface between cement and cancellous bone and furthermore an even, non-deficient cement mantle. A minimum cement mantle thickness of 2–3 mm is regarded essential to minimize the risk of osteolysis and loosening. Cement mantle thickness depends on femoral anatomy, stem size and design and centralizer usage. The radiographic results from a cadaver study suggest that critical zones of cement mantle thickness exist in Gruen zones 8/9 and 12, which can only be assessed on lateral radiographs. Cement penetration is improved by the use of a distal femoral plug, cement pressurizing techniques and pulsatile lavage, which have all been shown to reduce the risk of aseptic loosening. The influence of bone preparation, lavage technique and mode of cement application were investigated and the results are presented. Our findings indicate that syringe-lavage is significantly less effective with regard to cleansing capacity of cancellous bone as measured by cement penetration. Although pressurized application of cement is beneficial to improve cement interdigitation, thromboembolic complications may result as a consequence of raised intramedullary pressure. A new animal model is presented that confirms the efficacy of pulsatile lavage in reducing the bulk of medullary content. The use of pulsatile lavage (jet-lavage) is considered of paramount importance to achieve excellent cement penetration and to reduce the risk of fat embolism. Its use should be considered mandatory in cemented total hip arthroplasty.

Introduction

The pioneer of cemented total hip replacement (THR) Sir John Charnley created an amazingly high operative standard based on dedication and thorough basic research. His concept "low friction arthroplasty" still enjoys long-term success with Kaplan-Meier survival rates of 85–90% after 20 years [82, 119, 127, 145]. Other cemented stem designs showed a wide range between poor [3, 9, 132, 149, 151] and good results [22, 54, 66, 105, 106, 155] both clinically and radiographically. However, it soon became obvious, that not only stem design but in particular operative and cementing techniques had to be considered important factors influencing the outcome of cemented THR. Beckenbaugh and Ilstrup [9] found a strong correlation between poor packing of cement and radiographic loosening. The incidence of femoral loosening in well-seated and cemented components was only 5% within the alarmingly high 24% overall incidence 4–7 years postoperatively, which rose to 29.9% in a further follow-up study of the same patients after 10 years [149]. Using the same radiographic criteria Russotti et al. [141] reported a decrease of femoral loosening to 2.4% after 5–7 years using improved cementing techniques. Other studies have also shown higher rates of loosening when cement filling of the medullary canal was incomplete [90]. In this context several authors postulated a poor prognostic bearing of flaws and deficiencies in the cement mantle on the immediate postoperative radiograph [42, 72, 140].

Several clinical studies comparing patients before and after the introduction of modern cementing techniques have confirmed the benefit of improved cement application techniques [9, 22, 105, 106, 117, 140, 141, 149]; with the same benefit being found also in young patients [4, 7, 118]. Furthermore, if the risk for revision is taken as the measured outcome, the Swedish Hip Registry has provided important evidence to support this relationship [105, 106].

Cement–Bone Interface

When the first tissue from failed cemented prostheses became available for histological evaluation, bone necrosis and soft tissue at the cement-bone interface were noticed [163, 164]. It is of no surprise that bone cement was made responsible for the observed loosening phenomena and the term "cement disease" was coined [80]. Both animal [124] and post-mortem studies [164] have raised concern about the necrosis commonly seen at the junction between bone and cement. However, although bone necrosis will inevitably occur to some extent, Oates et al. [124] concluded from their study that the tissue damage may be offset by the benefit of improved fixation that cement pressurization techniques provide. Draenert [41] suggested that the formation of a fibrous membrane may not be intrinsic to the cementing process. In a rabbit model he described a true interface between bone and cement without the interposition of connective tissue. Similarly, in a dog model following cemented THA, direct bone to cement contact with bone apposition and good vascularization were demonstrated in the proximal, cancellous sections [131]. The authors attributed the absence of interface membrane formation to the use of modern cementing techniques; thus, achieving a secure mechanical interlock. However, in more distal sections, membranes were found to support the concept that poor mechanical fixation predisposes to connective tissue interposition at the interface. Thermal effects were considered unimportant for the occurrence of bone necrosis [131]. The maximum temperature before heat damage has to be contemplated seems to be in the area of 47 °C over a period of 1 min [50]. Sih et al. [147] showed that this temperature peak only occurs in pure cement mantles (without bone interposed) of greater than 3 mm thickness. If cancellous bone is present the maximum temperature in each cancellous compartment can be expected to be much lower, thus allowing deeper cement penetration without heat necrosis. In vivo studies would be helpful to confirm this assumption.

In the diaphyseal regions of a cemented implant where cancellous bone is sparse, the establishment of a sound mechanical interlock is more difficult. Surgical reaming that disrupts the diaphyseal blood supply may play an important role [131, 138]. A more complex remodeling response with formation of a secondary intramedullary cavity [41, 93] has to be contemplated. In contrast, the separate blood supply of proximal, metaphyseal cancellous bone gives an explanation as to why bone necrosis may not occur in the proximal area where mechanical interlock is best. This hypothesis is supported by the unique pattern of cement shrinkage within the trabeculae, which allows for rapid revascularization [14, 41]. A durable cement-bone interface has been documented in human post-mortem analysis of retrieved, well-fixed components up to 22 years following implantation [45, 78, 98, 107].

Preservation of Cancellous Bone

To achieve adequate cement interdigitation and a viable interlock, preservation of cancellous bone stock is of great importance. Although Charnley initially believed from his experience in fracture healing, that cancellous bone cannot carry the load [27], he later advocated preservation of cancellous bone for cemented anchorage [28]. "The cancellous structure can be regarded as a system of springs; the superficial layer of the cancellous bone in contact with the surface of the cement will *move as one* with the cement surface when load is applied; the deflection of the cancellous structure will take place inside the bulk of cancellous bone. In this way we can explain the paradox of the transmission of load from a hard to a soft substance without relative motion taking place between the surfaces in contact. It is on these grounds that I believe it is an advantage to have a layer of cancellous bone interposed between a cement surface and cortical bone." Based on his further clinical experience he later recommended preservation of 2–3 mm strong cancellous bone adjacent to the endosteal surface [29]. Draenert confirmed this view with his light- and electronmicroscopic findings in meticulous animal and post-mortem studies [14, 43, 46]. Preserved cancellous bone filled and stiffened with cement forms a viable construct/composite, which is resistant to deformation and is capable to carry the load [14, 46]. Numerous in vitro experiments have shown a strong correlation between improved cement penetration and increased shear strength of the cement-bone interface [2, 6, 60, 74, 88, 101, 103, 122, 130]. The interface strength is not only affected by the degree of cement penetration but also by the quality of the supporting cancellous framework [2, 9, 60].

This concept of creating a sound cement-bone construct is also supported by clinical and radiological experience. In a long-term radiographic study

Ebramzadeh et al. [48] discovered inferior outcome in cases where proximal cancellous bone had not been filled with cement. In conclusion they advocated removal of all medial cancellous bone. In contrast, Beckenbaugh and Ilstrup [9] had already pointed out that poorer outcome is not determined by preservation of bone, but due to failure to adequately "pack" the cement into proximal cancellous bone. In cases with poor proximal cement penetration a twofold increase in loosening rates had been observed [9].

The rigorous removal of cancellous bone was also suspected by Pellicci et al. [134] as a cause for failure. Less aggressive removal of cancellous bone has been associated with minimal femoral loosening rates after more than 10 years [126, 145]. In this context the poorer outcome of cemented femoral revisions [105] with deficient cancellous bone stock are of note and contradict the recommendation of removal of cancellous bone. Furthermore, cadaver studies [39] on the stability of the cement-bone interface in the revision scenario have provided convincing evidence supporting the concept of preservation of cancellous bone. After the first revision the interface shear strength was reduced dramatically to 20.6%, and decreased further to as little as 6.8% after the second revision compared to the primary situation.

Femoral Bone Preparation

To preserve cancellous bone stock careful femoral bone preparation is essential. Controversy exists regarding the optimal method of bone preparation for a cemented femoral stem [38]. DiGiannini et al. [38] reviewed the limited literature available on this subject and challenged the rationale and concept of the popular "ream and broach" preparation. It is indeed difficult to understand why destructive reamers should be inserted until the endosteal surface is hit. This intriguing maneuver removes cancellous bone thus creating a poor distal bone stock that is more similar to the revision situation. Reaming to cortex also increases the risk of bleeding by disrupting the arterial supply thus jeopardizing the establishment of a sound interface. Some laboratory studies have confirmed the detrimental effect of reamers on the shear strength of the cement-bone interface [5, 120] when compared with "broach only" techniques. Interestingly, limited research effort has been spent on the role of broach surface characteristics with regard to cement penetration. It has been suggested from in vitro studies [26] that in cemented femoral stems both cement penetration and primary stability are improved with bone compaction techniques using smooth tamps for canal preparation. However, it remains unclear whether jet-lavage had been used in this study. If no bone lavage was used, it is difficult to imagine why better cement penetration should occur in the presence of debris within the cancellous spaces. Furthermore, the sections presented in that study were not taken at the same level, so a valid conclusion regarding cement penetration cannot be drawn. Impaction of bone debris, which seems to be beneficial for cementless fixation [58], may contribute to primary stability in vitro. But this concept contradicts the proven advantages of lavaged bone with improved cement penetration and shear strength [6, 19, 21, 60, 88, 103].

Influence of Broach Surface upon Cement Penetration

Our own studies using a model with paired femora could not confirm the proposed advantage of compaction technique [18] with regard to cement penetration. In a cadaver study 29 paired human cadaver femora were prepared by using broaches of identical geometry but different surface characteristics. In one group of 24 pairs preparation with chipped-toothed broaches was compared with diamond-shaped broaches, in the other group of 9 pairs polished tamps for compaction of cancellous bone were compared with chipped-tooth broaches. Cancellous bone was irrigated with 1 litre saline by using pulsed lavage. The specimens were imbedded in specially designed pots (Fig. 1). Palacos R and Simplex bone cements were used. After vacuum mixing the cement was applied in a retrograde manner and subjected to a standard pressure protocol with a constant force of 3000 N. Horizontal sections were obtained at predefined levels using a diamond saw. Microradio-

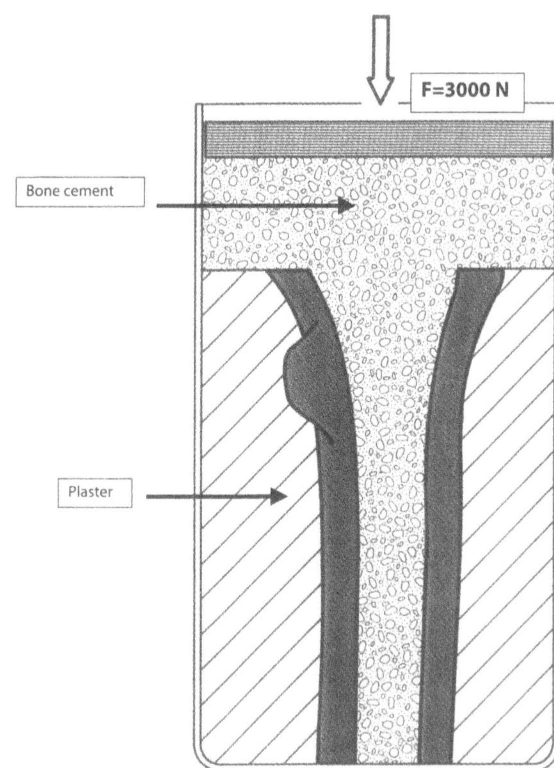

Fig. 1. Experimental configuration of a femur embedded in a canister using plaster of paris. Bone cement is placed in the femoral canal and up to the top of the canister. A 3000 N load is applied to the canister lid pressurizing the femoral canal in a controlled manner allowing for standardized cement pressurization

graphs were taken and analyzed to assess cement penetration into cancellous bone.

In 6 of 9 femora prepared by using smooth tamps fissures/fractures occurred despite careful preparation technique. The microradiographic evaluation revealed no significant morphometric differences in the different groups with regard to cement penetration into cancellous bone. These findings were similar in all sections obtained. Also, no significant difference was found between diamond broaching and chipped-tooth-canal preparation in the presence of thorough, standardized pulsatile lavage (Figs. 2, 3).

A previous study [14, 15] has shown, that significant destruction of the adjacent trabeculae can occur when blunt chipped tooth broaches of maximum size were inserted [14, 15, 46]. Fortunately, removal of cancellous bone

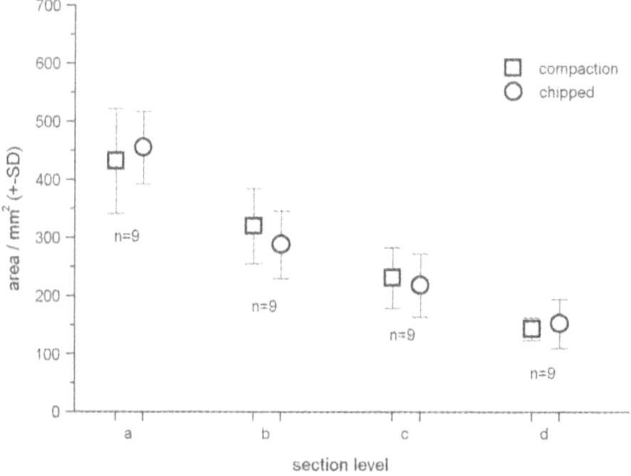

Fig. 2. Comparison of cement penetration in sections a–d for compaction (polished) and chipped tooth specimens

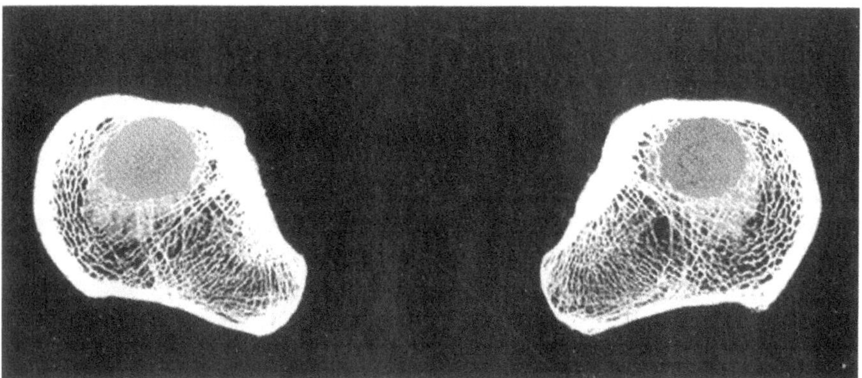

Fig. 3. Microradiographs. Cement penetration for matched femoral pairs broached using either a chipped or diamond tooth broach taken at the level of the lesser trochanter. There was no significant difference between broach type with regard to cement penetration

in the curved femur is almost never complete, which may offer an explanation why the published clinical results do not reveal a distinct difference between "ream and broach" and "broach only" techniques. A less traumatic method of bone preparation and preservation can be achieved using diamond wet-grinders [46], but no clinical results are available to support the theoretical advantage of this technique.

Although "broach only" techniques seem preferable and may be regarded as the "gold standard", careful bone sparing techniques should be implemented with whatever technique or instruments used.

Modern Cementing Techniques

Modern cementing techniques aim to improve the mechanical interlock between bone and cement in order to establish a durable interface. Cement interdigitation not only depends on bone preparation, but also on lavage and mode of cement application. Thorough cleansing of the bone bed by the use of jet-lavage, the use of a distal intramedullary plug and a proximal seal (representing second generation cement techniques) reduce the risk for revision by approximately 20% each [106]. With increased depth of cement penetration the strength of the cement-bone interface is enhanced [2, 60, 88, 130]. Both pressurization and lavage of cancellous bone have been identified to be significant factors with regard to improved cement penetration and, as a consequence, improved shear strength [2, 6, 19, 60, 88, 103, 109, 122, 130].

Bone Lavage

Halawa et al. [60] demonstrated the significance of bone quality and bone lavage prior to cementation with regard to improved mechanical shear strength. Krause et al. [88] observed in human tibias that the depth of bone cleaning by using lavage had a tendency to limit the depth of cement penetration. Bannister and Miles [6] had also found improved cement penetration and increased interface strength when bone lavage was used.

To our knowledge, it is common practice to use some form of lavage prior to cement application. However, only a few studies have concentrated on the effectiveness of the lavage type. Krause et al. [88] reported improved cement penetration and shear strength when high intensity lavage was used. Majkowski et al. [103] evaluated the effect of bone surface preparation upon cement penetration using slices of bovine bone. They found no difference between continuous and pulsed pressurized lavage and no further beneficial effect of brushing.

Although the benefit of pulsatile lavage has been documented both experimentally [21, 60, 102, 103] and clinically [105], national surveys in the United Kingdom [65] and Germany [16] have elucidated a low prevalence of pressurized jet-lavage in cemented THA. Syringe-lavage is often used as an alternative. Maistrelli et al. [102] compared jet-lavage versus syringe-lavage in human tibial specimens obtained at total knee arthroplasty and found significantly better penetration in the jet-lavage group. However, the authors only commented on the time of lavage but not on the amount of irrigation used. Therefore, it remains unclear whether volume or lavage quality is the more important factor.

Jet-Lavage Versus Syringe Lavage

We performed a study to compare the effectiveness of both jet- and syringe-lavage with regard to their cleansing capabilities as measured by cement penetration [21]. Sixteen paired human cadaver femora were prepared using conventional broaches. Cancellous bone was irrigated with 1 litre pulsed lavage in one femur and with 1 l syringe-lavage in the contralateral femur. The specimens were imbedded in specially designed pots (Fig. 1) and vacuum mixed bone cements were applied in a retrograde manner. After application of a standard pressure to the pots, the femurs were removed, radiographed and horizontal sections were obtained and analyzed to assess cement penetration. Our results show that in equal quality bone, the use of jet-lavage yields significantly ($P<0.0001$) improved rates of cement penetration compared to syringe-lavage specimens (Figs. 4, 5).

It is important to distinguish between various lavage types and volumes. We used identical irrigation volumes in our model to identify the effect of irrigation type rather than total volume. Furthermore, we used entire paired human femora and not bone slices to allow assessment of the entire femoral architecture. It was concluded that the use of high-volume pressurized jet-lavage for cleaning of the intramedullary cavity prior to cement application in THR should be routinely used in cemented total hip arthroplasty.

Pressurized Cement Application

The introduction of a distal intramedullary cement restrictor allowed for cement containment and pressurization resulting in improved cement penetration [74, 109] and better clinical outcome [62, 63, 117]. Charnley [28] had already emphasized the importance of achieving adequate cement pressure: "The cement is forced down the track of the medullary canal as a stiff dough and the insertion of the point of the tapered stem of the prosthesis expands the stiff dough and injects it into the cancellous lining of the marrow space..." Markolf and Amstutz [109] demonstrated that high proximal pressures (and improved cement penetration) occur proximally during "finger packing", the method introduced and advocated by Charnley [28, 29]. These pressures were comparable to peak pressure during prosthesis insertion. In contrast, Song et al. [148] had measured the highest intramedullar pressures during stem insertion and postulated that additional, prior cement impaction is probably unnecessary. Although McCaskie et al. [113] reported similar findings from their in vivo and additional laboratory studies, they did not

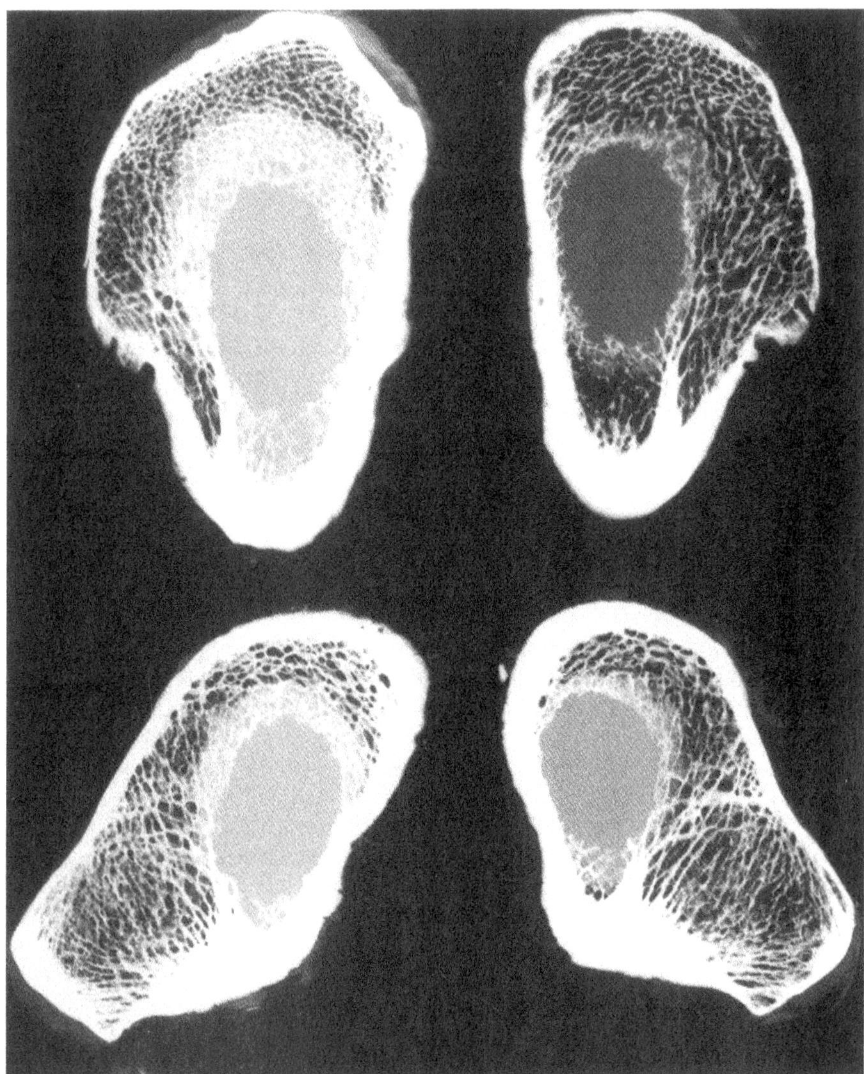

Fig. 4. Microradiographs. Cement penetration for jet-lavage and syringe lavage sections taken at the level of the lesser trochanter. Cement penetration increased in all specimens with jet-lavage (*left*) compared to the syringe-lavage specimens (*right*)

agree that stem insertion is the most significant part of cementing. However, it is not only the maximum peak pressures that determine cement penetration but also the time this pressure is maintained. The use of "sustained pressurization" provides increased cement penetration [8] and has been recommended by the Exeter group [94]. This technique is of particular importance when low viscosity cements are used to minimize the risk of blood laminations and weakening of the cement-bone interface [10, 104]. Results of

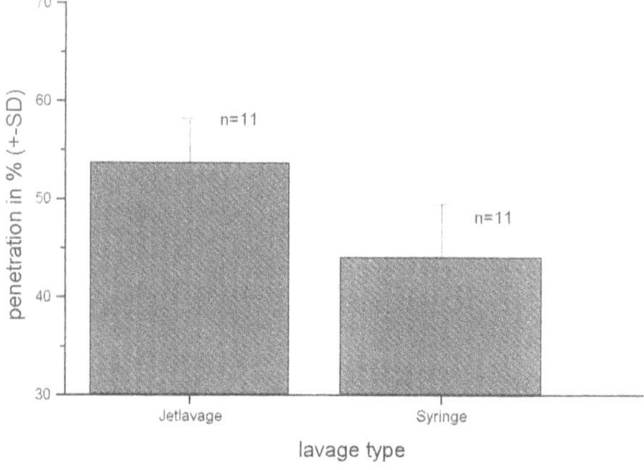

Fig. 5. Jet-lavage versus syringe lavage: comparison of cement penetration of paired femora where Palacos was used

in vitro studies [2, 10] demonstrated that 4–5 s duration of sustained pressure is probably sufficient to achieve most of the maximum cement penetration. Bleeding models have however suggested minimum periods of 30 s to be necessary to prevent blood entrapment and to obtain a satisfactory cementing result [2, 10]. Hypotensive anesthetic methods including epidurals, as well as the use of suction catheters and local hemostatic agents, e.g. H_2O_2 are also considered important and useful to reduce the amount of interface bleeding [111].

McCaskie et al. [113] provided good evidence that retrograde cement application generated higher cement pressures distally than proximally, a pattern reversed by finger packing. A proximal femoral cement compactor [125] further increases proximal cement pressures (and cement penetration), but pressurized cement fixation remains a demanding, time consuming and user-dependent procedure [159].

Although pressure measurements provide important information about the various steps of femoral cement application, the situation remains very complex and only evaluation of cement penetration can help to clarify the value and impact of the particular variables [113].

Impact of Lavage and Pressurizing

To determine the influence of jet-lavage and cement pressurizing techniques upon cement penetration into proximal femoral cancellous bone 60 left human cadaver femora were used for implantation of cemented stem components [19]. Four different groups of cementing techniques were generated (Fig. 6), the allocation into the groups was randomized. Bone lavage was carried out either using jet-lavage or manual syringe lavage, cement application differed with regard to the amount of pressurization used. Five different stem designs were used. Radiographs were taken and horizontal sections were obtained at predefined levels (2 cm) using a diamond saw. Microradiographs were taken and analyzed using image analysis to assess cement penetration into cancellous bone.

Both jet-lavage and pressurization of bone cement significantly improved the penetration of cement into cancellous bone ($P = 0.027$ and $P = 0.003$, respectively, Fig. 7). Stem insertion alone without additional pressurization during retrograde gun application and proximal packing resulted in inferior rates of cement penetration. In the presence of strong, dense cancellous bone the findings were more pronounced. An influence of the stem type upon outcome (penetration) was not observed. The results raise doubt whether adequate cement penetration can be achieved during stem insertion alone. It was concluded that high pressurizing techniques are an effective means of improving the interdigitation between cancellous bone and cement, but should only be administered in combination with jet-lavage to reduce the risk of thromboembolic complications.

These results and the evidence outlined above stress the clinical bearing of adequate proximal cement intrusion and may offer an explanation as to why excellent long-term results have been achieved with so-called first generation cementing techniques. However, there is no doubt that second generation techniques further improve cement penetration and as a consequence long-term outcome. Currently, these techniques have to be considered as "gold standard" [16, 65, 105, 111]. Whether "third generation" techniques with the use of modern cement preparation, new stem designs (e.g. precoating) and centralizer will lead to a further reduction of loosening rates remains to be seen.

Cementing technique	Lavage	Pressurised cement application	Digital pressurisation after cementation	Stem insertion using sustained pressure
A	Jet-Lavage	No	No	No
B	Jet-Lavage	Yes	No	Yes
C	Jet-Lavage	Yes	Yes	Yes
D	Syringe	Yes	yes	Yes

Fig. 6. Four different cementing techniques. Note that groups A–C differed with regard to the degree of pressurisation techniques. In groups C and D the same pressurization protocol was implemented, but lavage type differed

Group	Better penetration	Significance level	Factor
A versus B	B	$P = 0.024$	Pressure
A versus C	C	$P = 0.001$	Pressure
B versus C	C	$P = 0.360$	Pressure
C versus D	C	$P = 0.027$	Jet-Lavage

Fig. 7. Comparison of the different cementing techniques used. Note that groups A–C differed with regard to the degree of pressurization techniques. In groups C and D the same pressurization protocol was implemented, but lavage type differed

"Optimal" Cement Mantle Thickness

There is little doubt that a deficient cement mantle may be detrimental with regard to long-term implant survival. Thin layers of cement have less potential for energy absorption and may crack and fail [71, 92], in particular in the proximal and distal portions of the cement mantle [84]. Cement mantle fractures, localized osteolysis [25, 70, 108] and granuloma formation at the interface [1, 133] or failure [9, 128] may result as a consequence of direct implant to bone contact or very thin cement mantles around the stem tip [56, 128]. Furthermore, deficient cement mantles create a pathway for particulate wear debris to migrate along the stem-cement interface down to the cement-bone interface, thus initiating or accelerating particle-induced osteolysis and loosening [69, 77]. In contrast, complete cement mantles with a minimum thickness of 2–3 mm have been reported to be associated with better long-term radiographic outcome [48, 81, 82]. A clear distinction between pure cement mantles and cement mantles containing interdigitated cancellous bone has not been made and is difficult to attempt using plain radiographs. The adequacy of radiographic interpretation is subject to debate. Poor inter- and intraobserver reproducibility of radiographic cement mantle assessment have been reported [64, 85, 87, 112]. Cement mantle defects and the prevalence of thin cement mantles may be underestimated on routine radiographic assessment [75]. Cadaver studies have shown a poor correlation between radiographic and microradiographic assessment of the cement-bone interface [75, 137].

Although it is not justified to define an ideal cement mantle thickness, a minimum cement mantle thickness of 2 mm is widely accepted based on experimental and radiographic experience [2, 12, 48, 71, 82, 92, 94, 134, 144].

Femoral Configuration, Stem Design and Centralizer

The cement mantle thickness depends on stem design, size and shape as well as femoral geometry [15, 17, 35]. Anatomy and stem shape are beyond the surgeon's control, but stem size and stem design selection are the surgeon's responsibility. Large stem sizes implanted as "cemented press-fit" stems carry the risk of cement mantle deficiencies [15, 43] and may be associated with increased loosening rates [89, 110, 115]. Krismer et al. [89] reported a revision rate of 1.9% after 6–8 years for Müller straight (cemented press-fit) stems, but considered another 20.1% radiographically at risk. Oversizing of the stem resulting in incomplete cement mantles has also been suggested to account for early femoral component loosening in Chinese patients with small femora [30]. This observation is supported by the finite-element model of Lee et al. [95] and the biomechanical testing of Fisher et al. [52]. Similar to Huddleston [70] they concluded that · smaller stem sizes and not over-broaching are desirable to accomplish a favorable cement mantle thickness.

Results with Müller straight stems implanted using modern cementing techniques, where smaller stem sizes have probably been used to respect a minimum cement mantle thickness, are not dissimilar from results with other stem designs (Charnley, Exeter, Stanmore) [105, 106]. Interestingly, excellent results have been achieved using the anatomically adapted SPII prosthesis [1–6], which carries a low risk of thin cement mantles [15].

Influence of Stem Design and Centralizer

To study the influence of stem design, centralizer and femur type upon cement mantle thickness we performed a standardized cadaver study [17] on 48 left femora with four different stem designs (1 anatomic, 3 straight). A radiographic and microradiographic analysis was done. Overall 88% of stems were aligned within 1° of neutral in the frontal plane. In total 24 thin cement mantles (less than 2 mm) were determined in 19 specimens in Gruen zones 1 through 7 with no correlation to stem design or zone. In the sagittal plane typical areas of thin cement mantles were identified (Fig. 8) in Gruen zones 8 and 9 ($n=39$) and 12 ($n=21$). The anatomic stem design carried the lowest risk (54%) of producing a thin cement mantle proximally in Gruen zones 8/9. The risk for straight stem designs was more than 90%. Straight stems without centralizer showed the highest risk of thin cement mantles in Gruen zone 12 (93%).

The assessment of the cement mantle and stem alignment is commonly done concentrating on standard AP radiographs [7, 48, 57, 70, 87, 112]. Our results suggest that lateral radiographs are essential to detect inadequate cement mantle thickness, which typically seem to occur antero-proximally in Gruen zones 8/9 and posterior-distally in Gruen zone 12, particularly when straight stems are used. Lower femoral neck osteotomies and removal of the posterior anatomical calcar femorale [46, 114] allow a more posterior canal entry and as a consequence better alignment of a straight stem is possible. Berger et al. [11] postulated that the distal anterior bowing of the femur predisposes to anterior cement mantle deficiencies when centralizers are not used. In contrast, we could find no evidence for this mechanism and our results suggest that it is the proximal anatomy (and bowing) of the S-shaped femur that affects stem alignment in the sagittal plane most. Centralizers were efficient to prevent thin cement mantles in zone 12 but had no effect proximally, a finding similar to Berger et al. [11]. The benefit of centralizers with regard to improved long-term outcome remains subject to debate [152]. Centralizers may adversely affect the peak strains around the stem tip [51]. Complications associated with the use of centralizers include dislodgment from the stem tip, void accumulation and fracture [11, 34, 57, 61, 123]. However, there is increasing evidence that distal centralizers are useful to achieve a neutral stem alignment thus preventing an unfavorable varus position [9, 11, 128].

Anatomic stems allow for more even cement mantles and minimize the risk of thin cement mantles without the use of centralizers and may be considered in the femur with marked proximal bowing. It is difficult to predict the clinical implications of these findings and we hesitate to conclude that

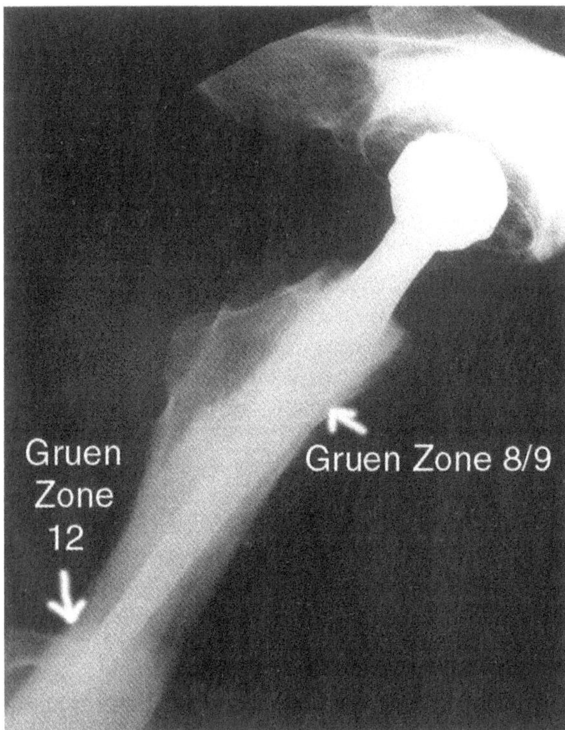

Fig. 8. Lateral postoperative radiograph following implantation of a straight cemented stem with a small centralizer. Despite posterior canal entry the stem shows an oblique orientation in the sagittal plane with critical areas of cement mantle thickness in Gruen zones 8/9 and 12

anatomical stems should be favored as a consequence. The clinical results from the Swedish hip registry [105, 106] were however excellent for an anatomic stem design at 13 years' follow-up in comparison with all other stems.

Stem Surface Characteristics

Not only stem geometry and centralizer, but also stem surface has to be considered as an important factor influencing survival of femoral components [116]. The experience from Exeter [54] and the results from the Swedish hip registry [105, 106] suggest that a highly polished surface may be more beneficial when straight stem designs are used allowing for subsidence within the cement mantle. A matte surface finish of stems with similar geometry was associated with higher failure rates [54, 105], Similarly, Dall et al. [36] reported marginally better results for polished flat-back Charnley stems than with the subsequent matte surface design. Fornasier and Cameron [53] observed a gap between stem and cement that was filled with a thin layer of connective tissue in human retrievals. This finding suggested micromovement and no rigid fixation of the prostheses to the cement. At the time the authors were uncertain of the clinical significance of their finding. In an attempt to strengthen the stem-cement interface "precoating" of the prosthesis was introduced. However, early clinical failures with debonding of the stem from the cement column resulted in the need for revision surgery [40]. The authors postulated that strengthening of the cement-prosthesis interface may magnify the deleterious effects of a poor cement mantle and predisposes this interface to failure. The same failure mechanism and a pattern of progressive loosening was described for another stem design [116] emphasizing the detrimental effect of roughening of the stem surface. If debonding occurs rapid cement abrasion can occur secondary to micromovement at the cement-stem interface. As a consequence from a finite element analysis Verdonschot et al. [156] concluded that debonded stems should either have a macrostructure to minimize micromotion or a polished surface to minimize the risk of cement abrasion. If one assumes from the evidence outlined above, that all cemented stems – regardless of surface characteristics – eventually debond because this interface cannot be maintained as a result of micromovement (at the cement-prosthesis interface), then only a smooth or polished surface could prevent cement abrasion and secondary induced particle/wear disease [142].

Although more and more evidence emerges supporting this hypothesis, it is currently not justified to condemn all non-polished surfaces, as some matte stem designs enjoy excellent clinical results [67, 105].

Stem material and cement mantle thickness may also play an important role in this context. Titanium has been blamed for some catastrophic early results [110] and is often regarded as an unsuitable material for cemented components. A rough titanium surface and a thin cement mantle have probably contributed significantly to the failure pattern of the Capital hip. In contrast, excellent clinical results – comparable to stainless steal components – have been achieved with non-rough titanium stems [67, 68]. Little is known about the relationship of stem material and ideal cement mantle thickness. It could well be that thinner cement mantles can be tolerated with (polished) titanium stems because of the lower elastic modulus compared to stainless steel. If this assumption is correct, even thicker cement mantles would be required if cobalt-chrome stems are used.

More research is needed to understand these complexities, in particular when the creep characteristics of bone cement are considered.

Bone Cement and Porosity Reduction

Failure and loosening of a cemented implant may be associated with poor biomechanical properties of bone cement and can also occur within the cement mantle itself [79, 149]. Large voids and flaws within the cement may lead to cement mantle fractures via a mechanism of rapid crack propagation [76]. Macroporosity has been shown to correlate with reduced fatigue strength and mechanical failure [76, 91]. Reduction of cement porosity is therefore a logical step in the attempt to improve the quality and fatigue life of cement. Improved biomechanical properties and reduced porosity can be achieved with cement centrifugation [23, 165] but antibiotics and radiopaque agents may not be intermixed evenly [37]. Vacuum mixing has been shown to be effective in achieving these objectives in vitro [97, 166], in particular in reducing microporosity [97, 158, 166]. The clinical relevance of microporosity reduction, however, remains subject to debate [96, 99, 139].

A satisfactory reduction of macroporosity, however, may not be achieved with vacuum mixing [97, 166], unless not only mixing but also collection of the cement is done under vacuum [157]. Wang et al. [158] have demonstrated that not all vacuum systems are equally effective in reducing the number and size of large voids. The "ideal" porosity has not yet been defined but Hahn et al. [59] postulated that beyond 3–5% porosity a further reduction may not be possible. The recent results from the Swedish national hip registry [106] have supported the proposed clinical benefit of vacuum mixing with a demonstrated reduction in the revision risk for loosening.

Low Viscosity Versus High Viscosity Cements

Certain types of bone cements seem to be more prone to failure [55, 66, 121]. The statistical data from the Swedish [106] and Norwegian hip registries [66] have shown better long-term outcome when high/normal viscosity cements (Palacos® and Simplex®) were used. In contrast, the use of low viscosity cements (CMW 3® and Boneloc®) was associated with a significantly higher risk of revision [66]. This finding seems to contradict the evidence from the basic science to some extent. Low viscosity cements were advocated due to their favorable flow characteristics [109].

In contrast to other authors [101], Simplex® has been categorized as high viscosity cement in the Scandinavian registries. Interestingly, if one looks carefully at the various experiments conducted with this cement, it becomes obvious that the time of cement application varies dramatically from study to study [8, 60, 88, 102, 104, 150]. Low viscosity cements have shown increased rates of cement penetration [47] and interface strength [60, 101, 150] in non-bleeding in vitro models. However, in the presence of active bleeding the interface shear strength with low viscosity cements is reduced dramatically [104], although the depth of cement penetration seems not to be affected to the same extent. Benjamin et al. [10] have demonstrated the detrimental effect of bleeding on the integrity of the cement-bone interface. The use of sustained pressure until the cement viscosity had increased to resist the displacement caused by the bleeding pressure was found essential when cement is injected in a low viscosity state. In the presence of bleeding bone the cementing technique with low viscosity cement may not be reliably reproducible [6]. Bannister and Miles [6] concluded from their experiments that low viscosity cement is the least important factor affecting interface strength. Similarly, Majkowski [104] found the rate of cement penetration to be determined more by morphology of cancellous bone rather than cement viscosity. In contrast, cement of higher viscosity is less susceptible to contamination with bleeding but must not be applied too late – otherwise the extent of penetration may be jeopardized [104]. From their finding in the bleeding situation Majkowski et al. [104] recommended meticulous pulsed lavage, rapid application of normal viscosity cement in the doughy state and immediate manual pressurization for at least 30 s.

In the clinical setting the clear distinction between low and high viscosity cement brands seems difficult. All cements pass through various phases of increasing viscosity during polymerization, so the timing of application remains the most decisive factor and all results published have to be interpreted with care. It is possible that if low viscosity cements are applied in a doughy state or in case of early insertion pressurization is maintained until a higher viscosity is reached, that results could equal the excellent outcomes reported with cements of higher viscosity [66], which seem more forgiving.

Fat Embolism

Cement pressurization causes a significant increase in intramedullary pressure (IMP) [49, 113, 143, 148]. As a consequence, fat and bone marrow embolization may result [13, 24, 83, 129, 153, 161]. The close relationship between raised IMP and cardio-respiratory complications has been well-established both experimentally [129, 153, 161, 162] and clinically [31–33, 135]. The rise of IMP has been recognized as the most decisive pathophysiological mechanism for the development of intraoperative embolism [160].

Cemented THR seems to be more prone to be associated with this phenomenon than cementless stem implantation [31, 68, 73, 129, 136]. The influence of the method of femoral cement application in this context has recently received increasing attention. Pitto et al. [135] found in their comparative study a substantial reduction of intraoperative embolism and cardio-respiratory impairment with the use of the so-called vacuum cementing technique [14, 44], which provides sufficient drainage of the medullary cavity during cementation via two cannulated screws. This new method of cement application is based on the finding that the main draining mechanism of the femur is along the linea aspera [44]. The clinical importance and benefit of a distal femoral venting hole as elaborated previously [13, 83, 153, 154]. However, a distal venting hole, which is not cleaned from bone cement, cannot heal (and remodel) and may act as a stress riser for femoral fractures.

Apart from creating an effective means of intramedullary drainage, thorough lavage with removal of medullary contents prior to cement application is an important logical step to reduce the risk of fat and bone marrow extravasations [146].

The beneficial role of pulsatile lavage by reducing medullary fat and bone marrow content in this context has been established both experimentally [20, 24, 146] and clinically [33]. Sherman et al. [146] demonstrated the benefit of thorough lavage by using a dog model. The significant decreases in arterial PO_2, increases in intrapulmonary shunt fraction and pulmonary artery pressure that had been evident in a non-lavage group were eliminated in the group having received thorough lavage. Similarly, Wheelwright et al. [162] studied cardiovascular effects of pulsatile lavage compared with non-lavage in a cemented arthroplasty dog model after cement and prosthesis insertion. They recorded severe hypotension, significant reduction in cardiac output with decreased systemic vascular resistance and elevated pulmonary artery pressure in the non-lavage group. Byrick et al. [24] had previously used a bilateral dog model to compare high-volume pulsatile lavage to low-volume manual lavage and found manual lavage insufficient to prevent pulmonary changes including microemboli. However, in their studies only one lavage type could be allocated per animal and no simultaneous cement application was done. Furthermore, cement application and stem insertion are difficult to reproduce in a standardized fashion. From the experimental evidence it remains unclear whether the lavage type or the irrigation volume is more value.

We performed a study [20] to directly compare the effectiveness of both pulsatile jet- and syringe-lavage with regard to their cleansing capabilities as measured by fat and bone marrow extravasation in a new sheep model allowing standardized bilateral, simultaneous cement pressurization. The operative procedure involved bilateral placement of intravenous catheters into the external iliac veins via retroperitoneal approaches. After femoral neck osteotomies both femoral cavities were prepared for retrograde cement application. After randomization one side was lavaged with 250 ml irrigation using a bladder syringe, the contralateral femur with the identical volume but using a pulsatile lavage. A specially designed apparatus was used to allow for bilateral simultaneous cement pressurization. Venous blood from both iliac catheters was then collected, anticoagulated and a quantitative fat analysis was performed.

Despite equal volume manual lavage produced significantly higher fat and bone marrow extravasation (Figs. 9, 10) than pulsatile lavage ($P<0.001$) thus suggesting that not only the volume but also the quality of bone lavage is an essential factor influencing the risk of fat embolism and adverse cardio-respiratory effects. Our findings further emphasize the important role of pulsatile lavage in preventing fat and bone marrow embolization during cemented total hip arthroplasty.

Interestingly, national surveys in the United Kingdom [65] and Germany [16] have elucidated a surprisingly low prevalence of pulsatile lavage in cemented THR. Syringe-lavage is often used as an alternative to jet-lavage, but fails to produce comparable rates of cement penetration [19, 21, 102] and puts the patient at a higher risk of fat embolic complications.

Sheep number	Pulsatile lavage	Syringe lavage	Ratio syringe to pulsatile
4	0.683	4.787	7.009
5	0.253	1.492	5.897
6	2.019	4.896	2.425
7	5.33	11.18	2.098
8	4.459	5.424	1.216
9	1.936	3.275	1.692
10	1.066	4.659	4.362
11	4.39	5.924	1.349
12	6.139	8.954	1.459
13	4.432	7.04	1.588
Sum	30.024	52.844	2.910
Mean	3.0707	5.7631	1.877
SD	2.111	2.762	

Fig. 9. Total fat intravasation per sheep (in grams), mean values and standard deviations (SD). The difference between pulsatile and syringe lavage was significant ($P<0.001$)

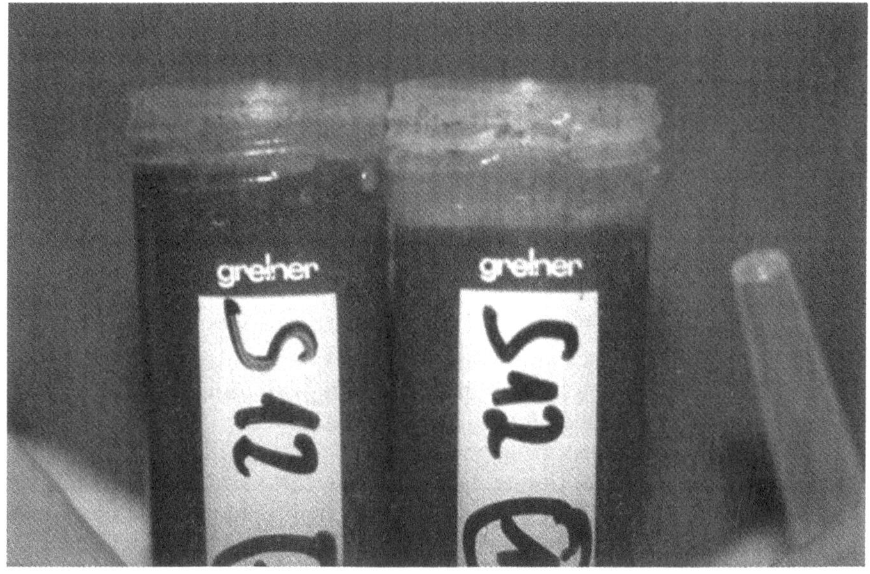

Fig. 10. Macroscopic appearance of blood samples collected. Note more supernatant fat on the blood surface in the syringe lavage group (*right*) than in pulsatile lavage group (*left*)

Author's Preferred Method

Based on the evidence outlined above the author describes his currently preferred method for cemented femoral arthroplasty:

1. Hypotensive anesthesia with epidural injection is preferred.
2. A posterior femoral canal entry is essential to minimize the risk of stem malalignment (in the sagittal plane) and cement mantle deficiencies.
3. A canal finder with a blunt distal section is used to preserve distal cancellous bone and arterial blood supply.
4. Prior to broaching, some proximal metaphyseal bone is removed using sharp U-shaped osteotomes/box osteotomes (or ideally diamond grinders).
5. A prominent posterior bone spike (i.e. the posterior extension of the femoral calcar) is resected prior to broaching.
6. Preoperatively templating is performed and a stem size allowing for a minimum cement mantle of 2–3 mm is selected. In doubt, down sizing of the stem is recommended.
7. Sharp broaches are used with the aim of preserving a rim of at least 3 mm cancellous bone medially. The broaches have to be kept in a posterior-lateral fashion.
8. Vacuum mixing of standard viscosity cement (prechilled Palacos® or other) is commenced. Usually two mixes of cement (80 g) are sufficient, but more cement can be necessary in large, stove-pipe femora.
9. Meticulous and copious high-pressure pulsatile lavage is performed to remove debris and marrow content. Usually 1 liter irrigation fluid is necessary.
10. A resorbable cement restrictor is inserted 1.5–2 cm distal to the expected tip of the prosthesis.
11. Lavage is repeated and the canal is packed with 3–5% H_2O_2-soaked ribbon gauze.
12. Suction tubing is placed allowing for intramedullary drainage during cement insertion.
13. At approximately 3–4 min (when Palacos® is used) after mixing the cement is applied via cement gun in a retrograde fashion using a proximal cement seal to allow for adequate pressurization.
14. Pressure is maintained for approximately 20–30 seconds.
15. Additional finger packing is performed to ensure further proximal cement penetration. (Note: If pressurization and cement penetration are adequate some fat extrusion can be observed at the proximal femur. In the routine case with reasonable cancellous bone stock interface bleeding ceases.)
16. At approximately 6 min a polished (anatomical) femoral component is slowly inserted by hand with a proximal seal in place until the stem has been seated 2/3 of its length. For the final insertion a loose fitting introducer is used. The insertion speed and pressure is balanced by the surgeon against the resistance from the cement. A hammer should not be used.

Conclusions

To perform a successful, long-lasting cemented THR, the surgeon needs to be prepared to strictly implement modern techniques of bone preparation, the use of pulsatile lavage and pressurization (or alternatively vacuum application) of cement. Performed well, this is a time-consuming procedure, which requires enthusiasm, dedication and perfectionism. If cementing technique is not perfect, the outcome may not be satisfactory both to the patient and the surgeon.

References

1. Anthony PP, Gie GA, Howie CR, Ling RSM (1990) Localised endosteal bone lysis in relation to the femoral components of cemented total hip arthroplasties. J Bone Joint Surg 72-B:971–979
2. Askew MJ, Steege JW, Lewis JL, Ranieri JR, Wixson RL (1984) Effect of cement pressure and bone strength on polymethylmethacrylate fixation. J Orthop Res 1:412–420
3. August AC, Aldam CH, Pynsent PB (1986) The McKee-Farrar hip arthroplasty: A long term study. J Bone Joint Surg 68-B:520–527
4. Ballard WT, Callaghan JJ, Sullivan PM, Johnston RC (1994) The results of improved cementing techniques for total hip arthroplasty in patients less than fifty years old. J Bone Joint Surg 76-A:959–964
5. Balu GR, Noble PC, Alexander JW, Vela VL (1994) The effect of intramedullary reaming on the strength of the cement/bone interface. Trans Orthop Res Soc 19:79
6. Bannister GC, Miles AW (1988) The influence of cementing technique and blood on the strength of the bone-cement interface. Eng Med 17:131–133
7. Barrack RL, Mulroy RD, Harris WH (1992) Improved cementing techniques and femoral component loosening in young patients with hip arthroplasty. J Bone Joint Surg 74-B:385–389
8. Bean DJ, Hollis JM, Woo SL-Y, Convery FR (1988) Sustained pressurization of polymethylmethacrylate: a comparison of low- and moderate viscosity bone cements. J Orthop Res 6:580–584
9. Beckenbaugh RD, Ilstrup DM (1978) Total hip arthroplasty. A review of three hundred and thirty-three cases with long follow-up. J Bone Joint Surg 60-A:306–313
10. Benjamin JB, Gie GA, Lee AJC, Ling RSM, Volz RG (1987) Cementing technique and the effect of bleeding. J Bone Joint Surg 69-B:620–624
11. Berger RA, Steel MJ, Wood K, Evans RN, D'Antonio J, Rubash HE (1997) Effect of a centralizing device on cement mantle deficiencies and initial prosthetic alignment in total hip arthroplasty. J Arthroplasty 12:434–443
12. Bocco F, Langan P, Charnley J (1977) Changes in the calcar femoris in relation to cement technology in total hip replacement. Clin Orthop 128:287–295
13. Breed AL (1974) Experimental production of vascular hypotension, and bone marrow and fat embolism with methylmethacrylate cement. Clin Orthop 102:227–244
14. Breusch SJ, Draenert K (1997) Vacuum application of bone cement in total hip arthroplasty. Hip International 7:1–16
15. Breusch SJ, Draenert Y, Draenert K (1998) Die anatomische Basis des zementierten Femurstieles. Eine Vergleichsstudie zum geraden und anatomischen Design. Z Orthop 136:554–559
16. Breusch SJ, Berghof R, Schneider U, Weiß G, Simank H-G, Lukoschek M, Ewerbeck V (1999) Der Stand der Zementiertechnik bei Hüfttotalendoprothesen in Deutschland. Z Orthop 137:101–107
17. Breusch SJ, Lukoschek M, Kreutzer J, Brocai DRC, Gruen T (2001) Cement mantle thickness dependency on femoral stem design and centralizer. J Arthroplasty (im Druck)
18. Breusch SJ, Norman TL, Revie IC, Lehner B, Caillouette JT, Schneider U, Blaha JD, Lukoschek M (2001) Cement penetration in the proximal femur does not depend on broach surface finish. Acta Orthop Scand (im Druck)

19. Breusch SJ, Schneider U, Kreutzer J, Ewerbeck V, Lukoschek M (2000) Einfluß der Zementiertechnik auf das Zementierergebnis am koxalen Femurende. Orthopäde 29:260–270
20. Breusch SJ, Reitzel T, Schneider U, Volkmann M, Ewerbeck V, Lukoschek M (2000) Zementierte Hüftendoprothetik: Verminderung des Fettembolierisikos in der zementierten Hüftendoprothetik mittels gepulster Druckspülung. Orthopäde 29:578–586
21. Breusch SJ, Norman TL, Schneider U, Reitzel T, Blaha JD, Lukoschek M (2000) Lavage technique in THA: jet-lavage produces better cement penetration than syringe-lavage in the proximal femur. J Arthroplasty 15(7):1–7
22. Britton AR, Murray DW, Bulstrode CJ, McPherson K, Denham RA (1996) Long-term comparison of Charnley and Stanmore design total hip replacements. J Bone Joint Surg 78-B:802–808
23. Burke DW, Gates EI, Harris WH (1984) Centrifugation as a method of improving tensile and fatigue properties of acrylic bone cement. J Bone Joint Surg 66 A:1265–1273
24. Byrick RJ, Bell RS, Kay JC, Waddell JP, Mullen JB (1989) High-volume, high pressure pulsatile lavage during cemented arthroplasty. J Bone Joint Surg 71-A:1331–1336
25. Carlsson ÅS, Gentz C-F, Linder L (1983) Localized bone resorption in the femur in mechanical failure of cemented total hip arthroplasties. Acta Orthop Scand 54:396–402
26. Chareancholvanich K, Bourgeault C, Loch D, Greer N, Lew W, Bechtold JE, Gustilo RB (1998) Stability of primary cemented femoral implants with compaction of autogenous cancellous bone. 65th AAOS, New Orleans
27. Charnley J (1957) The closed treatment of common fractures. E&S Livingstone, Edinburgh London
28. Charnley J (1970) Acrylic cement in orthopaedic surgery. E&S Livingstone, Edinburgh London
29. Charnley J (1979) Low friction arthroplasty of the hip: theory and practice. Springer, Berlin Heidelberg New York Tokyo
30. Chiu KH, Shen WY, Tsui HF, Chan KM (1997) Experience with primary Exeter total hip arthroplasty in patients with small femurs. J Arthroplasty 12:267–272
31. Christie J, Burnett R, Potts HR, Pell AC (1994) Echocardiography of transatrial embolism during cemented and uncemented hemiarthroplasty of the hip. J Bone Joint Surg 76-B:409–412
32. Christie J, Robinson CM, Pell AC, McBirnie J, Burnett R (1995) Transcardiac echocardiography during invasive intramedullary procedures. J Bone Joint Surg 77-B:450–455
33. Christie J, Robinson CM, Singer B, Ray DC (1995) Medullary lavage reduces embolic phenomena and cardiopulmonary changes during cemented hemiarthroplasty. J Bone Joint Surg 77-B:456–459
34. Collier MB, Noble PC, Kamaric E (1998) Accumulation of voids around distal centralizers in cemented total hip replacement. ORS, 44th Annual Meeting, New Orleans
35. Crawford RW, Psychoyios V, Gie G, Ling R, Murray D (1999) Incomplete cement mantles in the sagittal femoral plane: an anatomical explanation. Acta Orthop Scand 70:596–598
36. Dall DM, Learmonth ID, Solomon MI, Miles AW, Davenport JM (1993) Fracture and loosening of Charnley femoral stems. Comparison between first-generation and subsequent designs. J Bone Joint Surg 75-B:259–265
37. Dingeldein E, Wahlig H (1987) The effect of centrifugation on radiopaque materials and antibiotics admixed to bone cements. In: Draenert K, Rütt A (eds). Beiträge zur Implantatverankerung. Histomorph Bewegungsapp 3:105–110
38. DiGiovanni CW, Garvin KL, Pellicci PM (1999) Femoral preparation in cemented total hip arthroplasty: Reaming or broaching? JAAOS 7:349–357
39. Dohmae Y, Bechtold JE, Sherman RE, Puno RM, Gustilo RB (1988) Reduction in cement-bone interface shear strength between primary and revision arthroplasty. Clin Orthop 236:214–220
40. Dowd JE, Cha CW, Trakru S, Kim SY, Yang IH, Rubash HE (1998) Failure of total hip arthroplasty with a precoated prosthesis. 4- to 11-year results. Clin Orthop 355:123–136
41. Draenert K (1981) Histomorphology of the bone-to-cement interface: remodeling of the cortex and revascularization of the medullary canal in animal experiments. In: Salvati EA (ed) The hip proceedings of the ninth open scientific meeting of the HIP Society. The John Charnley Award Paper, CV Mosby, Saint Louis, pp 71–110
42. Draenert K (1986) Beobachtung zur Zementierung von Implantatkomponenten. Med Orthop Tech 106/6:200–205
43. Draenert K (1988) Zur Praxis der Zementverankerung. In: Forschung und Fortbildung in der Chirurgie des Bewegungsapparates 2. München: Art and Science

44. Draenert K (1989) Modern cementing techniques. An experimental study of vacuum insertion of bone cement. Acta Orthop Belg 55:273–293
45. Draenert K, Draenert Y (1992) Die Adaptation des Knochens an die Deformation durch Implantate. Strain-Adaptive Bone Remodelling. In: Forschung und Fortbildung in der Chirurgie des Bewegungsapparates 3. München: Art and Science
46. Draenert K, Draenert Y, Garde U, Ulrich Ch (1999) Manual of cementing technique. Springer, Berlin Heidelberg New York Tokyo
47. Dunne NJ, Orr JF (1998) Flow characteristics of curing polymethylmethacrylate bone cement. Proc Inst Mech Eng 212:199–207
48. Ebramzadeh E, Sarmiento A, McKellop HA, Llinas A, Gogan W (1994) The cement mantle in total hip arthroplasty. Analysis of long-term radiographic results. J Bone Joint Surg 76-A:77–87
49. Engela D, Beverland DE, Salvi V, Revie IC, Orr JF (1993) Pressure measurement in bone cement around hip replacement stems. Proceedings 6th Annual International Symposium on Custom Prosthesis, Florida
50. Eriksson RA, Albrektsson T (1984) Temperature threshold levels for heat-induced bone injury: a vital-microscopic study in the rabbit. J Prosthet Dent 50:101–107
51. Estok DM, Orr TE, Harris WH (1997) Factors affecting cement strains near the tip of a cemented femoral component. J Arthroplasty 12:40–48
52. Fisher DA, Tsang AC, Paydar N, Milionis S, Turner CH (1997) Cement-mantle thickness affects cement strains in total hip replacement. J Biomechanics 30:1173–1177
53. Fornasier VL, Cameron HU (1976) The femoral stem/cement interface in total hip replacement. Clin Orthop 116:248–252
54. Fowler JL, Gie G, Lee AJC, Ling RSM (1988) Experience with the Exeter total hip replacement since 1970. Orthop Clin North Am 19:477–489
55. Furnes O, Lie SA, Havelin LI, Vollset SE, Engesaeter LB (1997) Exeter and Charnley arthroplasties with Boneloc or high viscosity cement. Comparison of 1,127 arthroplasties followed for 5 years in the Norwegian Arthroplasty Register. Acta Orthop Scand 68:515–520
56. Garellick G (1998) On outcome assessment of total hip replacement. Thesis, Göteborg University
57. Goldberg BA, AL-Habbal G, Noble PC, Paravic M, Liebs TR, Tullos HS (1998) Proximal and distal femoral centralizers in modern cemented hip arthroplasty. Clin Orthop 349:163–173
58. Green JR, Nemzek DVM, Arnoczky SP, Johnson LL, Balas MS (1999) The effect of bone compaction on early fixation on porous-coated implants. J Arthroplasty 14:91–97
59. Hahn M, Engelbrecht E, Delling G (1990) Eine quantitative Analyse zur Bestimmung der Porosität von vorkomprimiertem und unter Vakuum gemischtem Knochenzement. Chirurg 61:512–517
60. Halawa M, Lee AJC, Ling RSM, Vangala SS (1978) The shear strength of trabecular bone from the femur, and some factors affecting the shear strength of the cement-bone interface. Arch Orthop Trauma Surg 92:19–30
61. Hanson PB, Walker RH (1995) Total hip arthroplasty cemented femoral component distal stem centralizer. J Arthroplasty 10/5:683–688
62. Harris WH, McGann WA (1986) Loosening of the femoral component after the use of the medullary-plug cementing technique. Follow-up note with a minimum five-year follow-up. J Bone Joint Surg 68-A:1064–1066
63. Harris WH, McCarthy JC, O'Neill DA (1982) Femoral component loosening using contemporary techniques of femoral cement fixation. J Bone Joint Surg 64-A:1063–1067
64. Harvey EJ, Tanzer M, Bobyn JD (1998) Femoral cement grading in total hip arthroplasty. J Arthroplasty 13:396–401
65. Hashemi-Nejad A, Goddard NJ, Birch NC (1994) Current attitudes to cementing techniques in British hip surgery. Ann R Coll Surg Engl 76:396–400
66. Havelin LI, Espehaug B, Lie SA, Engesæter LB, Furnes O, Vollset SE (2000) Prospective studies of hip prostheses and cements. A presentation of the Norwegian Arthroplasty Register 1987–1999. 67th Annual Meeting of the American Academy of Orthopaedic Surgeons, Orlando, March 15–19
67. Hinrichs F, Boudriot U, Griss P (2000) 10 year results with a cemented fine-grit-blasted titanium-aluminum-vanadium hip endoprosthesis shaft. Z Orthop 138:52–56
68. Hofmann S, Hopf R, Mayr G, Schlag G, Salzer M (1999) In vivo femoral intramedullary pressure during uncemented hip arthroplasty. Clin Orthop 360:136–146

69. Howie DW, Vernon-Roberts B, Oakshott R, Manthey B (1988) A rat model of resorption of bone at the cement-bone interface in the presence of polyethylene wear particles. J Bone Joint Surg 70-A:257–263
70. Huddleston HD (1988) Femoral lysis after cemented hip arthroplasty. J Arthroplasty 3:285–297
71. Huiskes R (1980) Some fundamental aspects of human joint replacement. Analyses of stresses and heat conduction in bone-prosthesis structures. Acta Orthop Scand [Suppl] 185:109–200
72. Ianotti JP, Balderston RA, Booth RE, Rothman RH, Cohn JC, Pikens GT (1986) Aseptic loosening after total hip arthroplasty. Incidence, clinical significance, and etiology. J Arthroplasty 1:99–107
73. Inadome T, Wall MC, Smith CL, Whiteside LA (1998) Femoral intramedullary pressure during in vitro cemented and cementless total hip arthroplasty. Orthop Trans 22:154–155
74. Indong OH, Carlson CE, Tomford WW, Harris WH (1978) Improved fixation of the femoral component after total hip replacement using a methacrylate intramedullary plug. J Bone Joint Surg 60-A:608–613
75. Jacobs ME, Koeweiden EMJ, Sloof TJJH, Huiskes R, van Horn JR (1989) Plain radiographs inadequate for evaluation of the cement-bone interface in the hip prosthesis. Acta Orthop Scand 60:541–543
76. James SP, Jasty M, Davies J, Piehler H (1992) A fractographic investigation of PMMA bone cement focusing on the relationship between porosity reduction and increased fatigue life. J Biomed Mater Res 26:651–662
77. Jasty MJ, Floyd WE, Schiller AL, Goldring SR, Harris WH (1986) Localized osteolysis in stable, non-septic total hip arthroplasty. J Bone Joint Surg 68-A:912–919
78. Jasty M, Maloney WJ, Bragdon CR, Haire T, Harris WH (1990) Histomorphological studies of the long-term skeletal responses to well fixed cemented femoral components. J Bone Joint Surg 72-A:1220–1229
79. Jasty M, Maloney WJ, Bragdon CR, O'Connor DO, Haire T, Harris WH (1991) The initiation of failure in cemented femoral components of hip arthroplasties. J Bone Joint Surg 73-B:551–558
80. Jones LC, Hungerford DS (1987) Cement disease. Clin Orthop 225:192–206
81. Joshi AB, Porter ML, Trail IA et al. (1993) Long-term results of Charnley low friction arthroplasty in young patients. J Bone Joint Surg 75-B:616–623
82. Joshi RP, Eftekhar NS, McMahon DJ, Nercessian OA (1998) Osteolysis after Charnley primary low-friction arthroplasty. A comparison of two matched paired groups. J Bone Joint Surg 80-B:585–590
83. Kallos T, Enis JE, Gollan F, Davis JH (1974) Intramedullary pressure and pulmonary embolism of femoral medullary contents in dogs during insertion of bone cement and a prosthesis. J Bone Joint Surg 56-A:1363–1367
84. Kawate K, Maloney WJ, Bragdon CR, Biggs SA, Jasty M, Harris WH (1998) Importance of a thin cement mantle. Autopsy studies of eight hips. Clin Orthop 355:70–76
85. Kelly AJ, Lee MB, Wong NS, Smith EJ, Learmonth ID (1996) Poor reproducibility in radiographic grading of femoral cementing technique in total hip arthroplasty. J Arthroplasty 11:525–528
86. Kerboull L, Courpied JP, Chamberlin B, Kerboull M (1998) Long term results of Charnley-Kerboull total hip replacement in patients younger than 40. European Hip Society, 3rd Congress. Beaune 25–27 June
87. Kramhoft M, Gehrchen PM, Bodther S, Wagner A, Jensen F (1996) Inter- and intraobserver study of radiographic assessment of cemented total hip arthroplasties. J Arthroplasty 11:272–276
88. Krause W, Krug W, Miller JE (1982) Strength of the cement-bone interface. Clin Orthop 163:290–299
89. Krismer M, Klar M, Klestil T, Frischhut B (1991) Aseptic loosening of straight- and curved-stem Müller femoral prostheses. Arch Orthop Trauma Surg 110:190–194
90. Kristiansen B, Jensen JS (1985) Biomechanical factors in loosening of the Stanmore hip. Acta Orthop Scand 56:21–24
91. Kurdy NM, Hodgkinson JP, Haynes R (1996) Acrylic bone-cement. Influence of mixer design and unmixed powder. J Arthroplasty 11:813–819
92. Kwak BM, Lim OK, Kim YY, Rim K (1979) An investigation of the effect of cement thickness on an implant by finite element analysis. Int Orthop 2:315–319
93. Kwong LM, Jasty M, Mulroy RD, Maloney WJ, Bragdon CR, Harris WH (1992) The histology of the radiolucent line. J Bone Joint Surg 74-B:76–73

94. Lee AJC, Ling RSM (1981) Improved cementing techniques. Am Acad Orthop Surg Instr Course Lect 30:407–413
95. Lee IY, Skinner HB, Keyak JH (1994) Effects of variation of prosthesis size on cement stress at the tip of a femoral implant. J Biomed Mat Res 28:1055–1060
96. Lewis G, Nyman J, Trieu HH (1998) The apparent fracture toughness of acrylic bone cement: effect of three variables. Biomaterials 19:961–967
97. Lidgren U, Drar H, Möller J (1984) Strength of polymethylmethacrylate increased by vacuum mixing. Acta Orthop Scand 55:536–541
98. Linder L, Hansson HA (1983) Ultrastructural aspects of the interface between bone and cement in man. Report of three cases. J Bone Joint Surg 65-B:646–649
99. Ling RSM (1998) Porosity reduction in cement is not necessary for cemented total hip arthroplasty. The Hip Society and AAHKS, New Orleans, p 22
100. Ling RS, Lee AJ (1998) Porosity reduction in acrylic cement is clinically irrelevant. Clin Orthop 355:249–253
101. MacDonald W, Swarts E, Beaver R (1993) Penetration and shear strength of cement-bone interfaces in vivo. Clin Orthop 286:283–288
102. Maistrelli GL, Antonelli L, Fornasier V, Mahomed N (1995) Cement penetration with pulsed lavage versus syringe lavage in total knee arthroplasty. Clin Orthop 312:261–265
103. Majkowski RS, Miles AW, Bannister GC, Perkins J, Taylor GJS (1993) Bone surface preparation in cemented joint replacement. J Bone Joint Surg 75-B:459–463
104. Majkowski RS, Bannister GC, Miles AW (1994) The effect of bleeding on the cement-bone interface. Clin Orthop 299:293–297
105. Malchau H, Herberts P (1998) Prognosis of total hip replacement in Sweden: Revision and re-revision rate in THR. Presented at the 65th Annual Meeting of the American Academy of Orthopaedic Surgeons, New Orleans
106. Malchau H, Herberts P, Söderman P, Odén A (2000) Prognosis of total hip replacement: Update and validation of results from the Swedish National Hip Arthroplasty Registry. 67th Annual Meeting of the American Academy of Orthopaedic Surgeons, Orlando, pp 15–19
107. Malcolm AJ (1990) Pathology of cemented low-friction arthroplasties in autopsy specimens. In: Older J (ed) Implant bone interface. Springer, Berlin Heidelberg New York Tokyo, pp 77–82
108. Maloney WJ, Jasty M, Rosenberg A, Harris WH (1990) Bone lysis in well-fixed cemented femoral components. J Bone Joint Surg 72-B:966–970
109. Markolf KL, Amstutz HC (1976) In vitro measurement of bone-acrylic interface pressure during femoral component insertion. Clin Orthop 121:60–66
110. Massoud SN, Hunter JB, Holdsworth BJ, Wallace WA, Juliusson R (1997) Early femoral loosening in one design of cemented hip replacement. J Bone Joint Surg 79-B:603–608
111. McCaskie AW, Gregg PJ (1994) Femoral cementing technique: current trends and future developments. J Bone Joint Surg 76B:176–177
112. McCaskie AW, Brown AR, Thompson JR, Gregg PJ (1996) Radiological evaluation of the interfaces after cemented total hip replacement. Interobserver and intraobserver agreement. J Bone Joint Surg 78-B:191–194
113. McCaskie AW, Barnes MR, Lin E, Harper WM, Gregg PJ (1997) Cement pressurisation during hip replacement. J Bone Joint Surg 79-B:379–384
114. Merkel F (1874) Betrachtungen über das Os femorale. Arch Path Anat LIXI:237–256
115. Möllenhoff G, Graf M, Walz M, Muhr G (1995) Die Grunderkrankung als prognostisch wichtiger Parameter bei der Beurteilung von Langzeitergebnissen von Totalendoprothesen des Hüftgelenkes anhand von 8- bis 10-Jahres-Ergebnissen der zementierten Totalendoprothese Müller-Geradschaft. Orthop Praxis 2:114–117
116. Mohler CG, Callaghan JJ, Collis DK, Johnston RC (1995) Early loosening of the femoral component at the cement-prosthesis interface after total hip replacement. J Bone Joint Surg 77-A:1315–1322
117. Mulroy RD, Harris WH (1990) The effect of improved cementing techniques on component loosening in total hip replacement. An 11-year radiographic review. J Bone Joint Surg 72-B:757–760
118. Mulroy RD, Harris WH (1997) Acetabular and femoral fixation 15 years after cemented total hip surgery. Clin Orthop 337:118–128
119. Neumann L, Freund KG, Sorensen KH (1994) Long-term results of Charnley total hip replacement. Review of 92 patients at 15 to 20 years. J Bone Joint Surg 76-B:245–251

120. Newman MA, Bargar WL, Hayes DEJr, Taylor JK (1993) Femoral canal preparation for cemented stems: reamers versus broaches. 60th Annual Meeting of the American Academy of Orthopaedic Surgeons, San Francisco
121. Nilsen AR, Wiig M (1996) Total hip arthroplasty with Boneloc: loosening in 102/157 cases after 0.5–3 years. Acta Orthop Scand 67:57–59
122. Noble PC, Espley AJ (1982) Examination of the influence of surgical technique upon the adequacy of cement fixation in the femur. J Bone Joint Surg 64-B:120–121
123. Noble PC, Collier MB, Maltry JA, Kamaric E, Tullos HS (1998) Pressurization and centralization enhance the quality and reproducibility of cement mantles. Clin Orthop 355:77–89
124. Oates KM, Barrera DL, Tucker WN, Chau CC, Bugbee WD, Convery FR (1995) In vivo effect of pressurization of polymethyl methacrylate bone-cement. Biomechanical and histologic analysis. J Arthroplasty 10:373–881
125. Oh I, Bourne RB, Harris WH (1983) The femoral cement compactor. An improvement in cementing technique in total hip replacement. J Bone Joint Surg 65-A:1335–1338
126. Older J (1986) Low friction arthroplasty of the hip, a 10–12-year follow-up study. Clin Orthop 211:36–42
127. Older J, Butorac R (1992) Charnley low friction arthroplasty (LFA): a 17–21 year follow-up study. J Bone Joint Surg 74-B [Suppl III]:251
128. Olsson SS, Jernberger A, Tryggö D (1981) Clinical and radiological long-term results after Charnley-Müller total hip replacement. Acta Orthop Scand 52:531–542
129. Orsini EC, Byrick RJ, Mullen JB, Kay JC, Waddell JP (1987) Cardiopulmonary function and pulmonary microemboli during arthroplasty using cemented or non-cemented components. The role of intramedullary pressure. J Bone Joint Surg [Am] 69:822–832
130. Panjabi MM, Cimino WR, Drinker H (1986) Effect of pressure on bone cement stiffness. Acta Orthop Scand 57:106–110
131. Paul HA, Bargar WL (1986) Histologic changes in the dog femur following total hip replacement with current cementing techniques. J Arthroplasty 1:5–9
132. Pavlov PW (1987) A 15 year follow-up study of 512 consecutive Charnley-Müller total hip replacements. J Arthroplasty 2:151
133. Pazzaglia UE (1990) Pathology of the bone-cement interface in loosening of total hip replacement. Arch Orthop Trauma Surg 109:83–88
134. Pellicci PM, Salvati EA, Robinson HJ (1979) Mechanical failures in total hip replacement requiring reoperation. J Bone Joint Surg 61-A:28–36
135. Pitto RP, Koessler M, Draenert K (1998) The John Charnley Award. Prophylaxis of fat and bone marrow embolism in cemented total hip arthroplasty. Clin Orthop 355:23–34
136. Pitto RP, Koessler M, Kuehle JW (1999) Comparison of fixation of the femoral component without cement and fixation with use of a bone-vacuum cementing technique for the prevention of fat embolism during total hip arthroplasty. A prospective, randomized clinical trial. J Bone Joint Surg Am 81:831–843
137. Reading AD, McCaskie AW, Gregg PJ (1999) The inadaequacy of standard radiographs in detecting flaws in the cement mantle. J Bone Joint Surg 81-B:167–170
138. Rhinelander FW, Nelson CL, Stewart RD, Stewart CL (1979) Experimental reaming of the proximal femur and acrylic cement implantation: vascular and histologic effects. Clin Orthop 141:74–89
139. Rimnac M, Wright TM, McGill D (1986) The effect of centrifugation on the fracture properties of acrylic bone cements. J Bone Joint Surg 68-A:281–287
140. Roberts DW, Poss R, Kelley K (1986) Radiographic comparison of cementing techniques in total hip arthroplasty. J Arthroplasty 1:241
141. Russotti GM, Coventry MB, Stauffer RN (1988) Cemented total hip arthroplasty with contemporary techniques. A five-year follow-up study. Clin Orthop 235:141–147
142. Sabokbar A, Pandey R, Quinn JM, Athanasou NA (1998) Osteoclastic differentiation by mononuclear phagocytes containing biomaterial particles. Arch Orthop Trauma Surg 117:136–140
143. Savage AP, Revie IC, Orr JF (1993) Pressure measurement in bone cement around hip replacement stems. Innov Technol Biol Med 14:4
144. Schmalzried TP, Harris WH (1993) Hybrid total hip replacement. A 6.5 year follow-up study. J Bone Joint Surg 75-B:608–615
145. Schulte KR, Callaghan JJ, Kelley SS, Johnston RC (1993) The outcome of Charnley total hip arthroplasty with cement after a minimum twenty-year follow-up. The results of one surgeon. J Bone Joint Surg 75-A:961–975

146. Sherman RM, Byrick RJ, Kay JC, Sullivan TR, Waddell JP (1983) The role of lavage in preventing hemodynamic and blood-gas changes during cemented arthroplasty. J Bone Joint Surg 65-A:500–506
147. Sih GC, Connelly GM, Berman AT (1980) The effect of thickness and pressure on the curing of PMMA bone cement for the total hip joint replacement. J Biomech 13:347–352
148. Song Y, Goodman SB, Jaffe RA (1994) An in vitro study of femoral intramedullary pressures during hip replacement using modern cement technique. Clin Orthop 302:297–304
149. Stauffer RN (1982) Ten year follow-up study of total hip replacement: with particular reference to roentgenographic loosening of the components. J Bone Joint Surg 64-A:983–990
150. Stone JJ-S, Rand JA, Chiu EK, Grabowski JJ, An K-N (1996) Cement viscosity affects the bone-cement interface in total hip arthroplasty. J Orthop Res 14:834–837
151. Sutherland CJ, Wilde AH, Borden LS, Marks KE (1982) A ten-year follow-up of one hundred consecutive Müller curved-stem total hip replacement arthroplasties. J Bone Joint Surg 64-A:970–982
152. Tolo ET, Wright JM, Bostrom MP-G, Pellicci P, Salvati EA (1998) The effect of two different types of distal centralizers on the cement mantle thickness and stem alignment in total hip arthroplasty. AAOS Annual Meeting, New Orleans
153. Tronzo RG, Kallos T, Wyche MQ (1974) Elevation of intramedullary pressure when methylmethacrylate is inserted in total hip arthroplasty. J Bone Joint Surg 56-A:714–718
154. Ulrich C (1995) Value of venting drilling for reduction of bone marrow spilling in cemented hip endoprosthesis. Orthopäde 24:138–143
155. Van der Schaaf DB, Deutman R, Mulder TJ (1988) Stanmore total hip replacement: A 9–10 year follow-up. J Bone Joint Surg 70-B:45
156. Verdonschot N, Tanck E, Huiskes R (1998) Effects of prosthesis surface roughness on the failure process of cemented hip implants after stem-cement debonding. J Biomed Mater Res 42:554–559
157. Wang JS, Franzen H, Jonsson E, Lidgren L (1993) Porosity of bone cement reduced by mixing and collecting under vacuum. Acta Orthop Scand 64:143–146
158. Wang JS, Toksvig-Larsen S, Muller-Wille P, Franzen H (1996) Is there any difference between vacuum mixing systems in reducing bone cement porosity? Biomed Mater Res 33:115–119
159. Weber BG (1988) Pressurized cement fixation in total hip arthroplasty. Clin Orthop 232:87–95
160. Wenda K, Degreif J, Runkel M, Ritter G (1993) Pathogenesis and prophylaxis of circulatory reactions during total hip replacement. Arch Orthop Trauma Surg 112:260–255
161. Wenda K, Lauer K, Boor S, Runkel M, Kreitner KF (1995) Is there a connection between intramedullary pressure increase, bone marrow intravasation and deep venous thrombosis of the leg in endoprosthetics? Orthopäde 24:114–122
162. Wheelwright EF, Byrick RJ, Wigglesworth DF (1993) Hypotension during cemented arthroplasty. Relationship to cardiac output and fat embolism. JBJS 75-B:715–723
163. Willert HG, Puls P (1972) Die Reaktion des Knochens auf Knochenzement bei der Allo-Arthroplastik der Hüfte. Arch Orthop Unfall Chir 72:33–71
164. Willert HG, Ludwig J, Semlitsch M (1974) Reaction of bone to methacrylate after hip arthroplasty: a long-term gross, light microscopic, and scanning electron microscopic study. J Bone Joint Surg 56-A:1368–1382
165. Wixson RL (1992) Do we need to vacuum mix or centrifuge cement? Clin Orthop 285:84–90
166. Wixson RL, Lautenschlager EP, Novak MA (1987) Vacuum mixing of acrylic bone cement. J Arthroplasty 2:141–149

Bone Cement Porosity in Vacuum Mixing Systems

JIAN-SHENG WANG, FRED KJELLSON

Introduction

It is believed that the porosity of orthopedic bone cement influences the long-term mechanical stability and thus survival of joint prostheses. Various studies have shown that pores within the cement are detrimental to the fatigue properties of bone cement and that removal of air inclusions can enhance the fatigue properties significantly [1–3]. Fractographic analyses of cement specimens have shown that the primary failures in vivo were remarkably similar to fatigue failures in vitro; the fractured surfaces contain large pores that lead to rapidly propagating cracks and subsequent cement fracture [4–6].

Currently the most popular cement mixing technique is mixing under vacuum, which has been used for over 15 years, initially for environment reasons. There is extensive evidence that vacuum mixing reduces cement porosity. This porosity reduction increases the static and fatigue mechanical strength of bone cement compared to hand-mixed cement [1, 7, 8]. Vacuum mixing also reduces the interface porosity between the cement and prosthesis [9, 10] and the number of cement particles not bonded with the bulk of the cement [11].

Despite efforts to improve cementing techniques for joint replacement, a variation in the quality of bone cement after mixing may nullify their use. It might be expected that all cements mixed under vacuum would have reduced porosity if other details were not considered. Kühn [12] has repeatedly emphasized that not all cements are alike and that the properties of cement are changed by even slight variations in composition. Also, the vacuum mixing systems have different vacuum levels and mixing methods. Thus, the actual cured cement may have variations in quality, for example porosity, which may influence substantially the long-term clinical results of joint replacement. Therefore, the factors that influence bone cement porosity in vacuum mixing systems are of interest.

General Methods of Cement Porosity Investigation

Bone Cement Mixing

We have investigated Palacos® R, Palamed®, Osteopal® (Merck Biomaterial GmbH, Darmstadt, Germany), Palacos® R (Schering Plough Corp., Kenilworth, N.J., USA), Simplex® P (Howmedica Inc., Rutherford, N.J., USA) and Osteobond® (Zimmer Inc., Warsaw, Ind., USA) cements in the different vacuum mixing tests. The vacuum mixing systems Cemvac® (Cemvac System AB, Linköping, Sweden), VCS® (Merck Biomaterial GmbH, Darmstadt, Germany), Mitvac® (Scandimed AB, Sjöbo, Sweden), Optivac® (Scandimed AB, Sjöbo, Sweden), Osteobond® (Zimmer Inc., Warsaw, Ind., USA), Stryker® (Stryker Instruments, Kalamazoo, Mich., USA) were used, in addition to experimental mixing systems. All cements were kept at room temperature (21–22 °C) before mixing, except Palacos® R which was pre-chilled to 4 °C, as advised by the manufacturer. All the cements were mixed at 21–22 °C with or without vacuum. The cement mixing methods were according to the manufacturers' recommendations. Six to ten mixtures (one, two, or three packages) were done in each group. All cement mixes were included in the analyses.

Bone Cement Porosity Analysis

Two types of pores have been widely classified in fully polymerized bone cement: macropores (pore diameter >1.0 mm) and micropores (pore diameter ≈ 0.1–1.0 mm) [2, 3, 13–15].

Macropores. After mixing, the cement was collected into nozzles ($\varnothing$ 9.5× 200 mm). Standardized radiographs (i.e., 50 kV, 16 mAs and 100 cm focus film distance) were taken of the cement cylinders in the nozzles. These radiographs were used to count the number of pores greater than 1 mm in diameter, and the sizes were measured using a microscope connected to an image-analyzing system (Videoplan system, Kontron Bild-Analyse GmbH, Germany).

Micropores. Five-millimeter thick cement slices from the middle of the cement cylinder were cut by a low-speed water-cooled diamond saw (Isomet, Bueler Corp., Germany). The surfaces of the slices were stained, enabling the dark-stained voids to be identified. The micropores were measured under the microscope with incident light (magnification ×5) and the number of micropores in the cross-section (78.5 mm^2) were counted.

Density. The slices from the cement cylinder were measured using an electronic balance with a density kit (AE 260 Mettler Instrument Corp., Greifensee, Switzerland).

Factors That Influence Bone Cement Porosity in Vacuum Mixing Systems

Vacuum Level

Alkire et al. [7] used high vacuum mixing as a method of reducing the porosity of bone cement. A nearly pore-free product could be achieved at about 0.05 bar. In our investigation [13], a high-viscosity cement, Palacos® R, was mixed in a Mitvac® vacuum mixing system at 1 bar (atmospheric pressure), 0.2 bar, and 0.05 bar. The number of macropores was reduced by about 50% from using vacuum mixing, and the density increased significantly compared to mixing at atmospheric pressure. There was no significant difference between the 0.2 bar and 0.05 bar pressure levels, but a tendency was observed to get larger diameter macropores at the 0.05 bar level compared to 0.2 bar (Table 1). The results indicated that the higher vacuum level (0.05 bar) did not decrease the macropores for a high-viscosity cement, whereas it may increase the size of pores (Fig. 1 A, sample c). However, when collection under vacuum is also performed there is a porosity reduction (see "Cement Collection").

Cement Collection

One of the advantages of the vacuum mixing system is reduced cement porosity. However, pores cannot always be avoided by using vacuum mixing. X-ray observation showed that large pores were trapped during collection of the high-viscosity cement after vacuum mixing (Fig. 2 A). An experimental study [13] was performed to reduce the porosity of bone cement by avoiding the entrapment of air during cement collection under vacuum. Palacos® R was mixed in an experimental system. After vacuum mixing, the vacuum was kept and the cement was slowly collected under vacuum until the cement was totally compacted and then injected into nozzles. The results (Table 1 and 2) showed that the number of macropores decreased from 1.0 to 0.2 cm^{-3} in low vacuum (0.2 bar) and disappeared at higher vacuum (0.05 bar) when using vacuum collection. This finding suggested that a continuous vacuum from mixing to cement collection avoids macropore entrapment in high viscosity cement (Fig. 2 B). When a higher vacuum level is used, the vacuum collection of cement will limit the formation of macropores as well as micropores (Fig. 1 A, B, sample c), which may ensure pore free cement.

Table 1. Number, size, and volume of macropores and density at different vacuum levels (median, range). (Data from Wang et al. [13])

Pressure (bar)	Number of macropores cm^{-3}	Macropore diameter (mm)	Macropore volume (%)	Density (g cm^{-3})
1	2.3 (1.6–3.0)	1.85 (1.77–1.90)	0.73 (0.51–0.69)	1.151 (1.093–1.213)
0.2	1.0 (0.6–1.8)	1.88 (1.18–2.52)	0.34 (0.06–0.95)	1.269 (1.259–1.277)
0.05	1.0 (0.2–1.7)	2.02 (1.68–3.14)	0.47 (0.15–1.30)	1.281 (1.265–1.285)

A

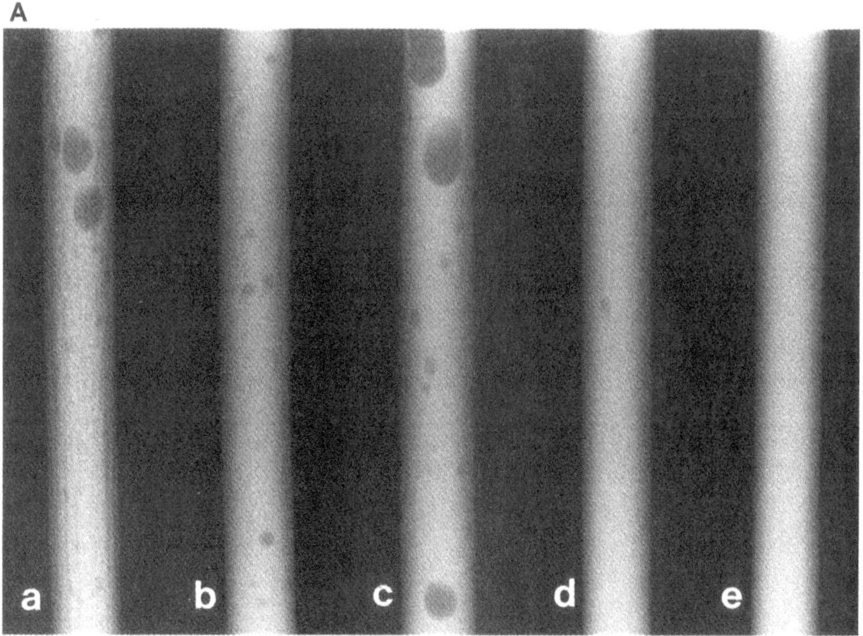

B

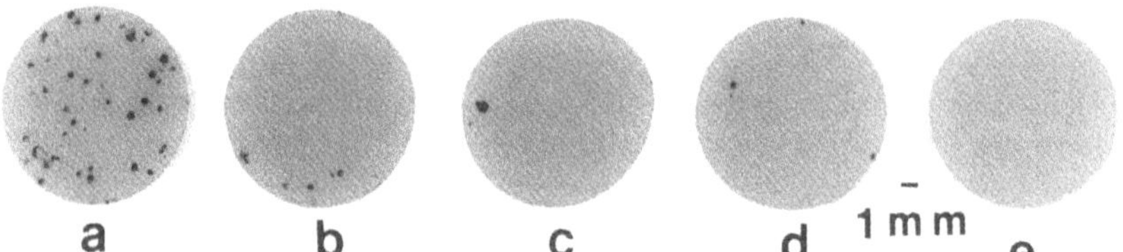

Fig. 1. A Radiograph of cement cylinders showing the macropores of the cement. **B** Cross sections showing the micropores of the cement. *a* Mixing at 1 bar (atmospheric pressure). *b* Mixing at 0.2 bar. *c* Mixing at 0.05 bar. *d* Mixing and collection at 0.2 bar. *e* Mixing and collection at 0.05 bar

Boiling of Monomer During Vacuum

Alkire et al. [7] suggested that the reduction of porosity was linked with increased vacuum level and a nearly pore-free product could be achieved at 0.05 bar [7, 13]. Wixson et al. [8] found that if a higher vacuum than 0.2 bar is used, the monomer tends to boil, possibly introducing more porosity into cement. They recommend a vacuum level range between 0.33 and 0.27 bar. We found that down to a vacuum level of 0.05 bar there was no obvious sign

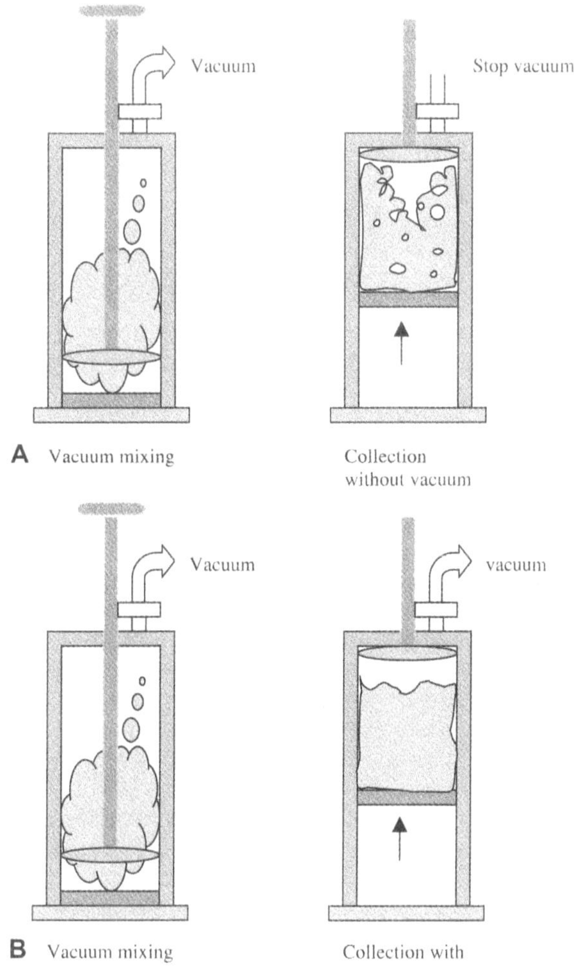

Fig. 2. Illustration showing air bubbles being trapped in cement during collection (**A**); this can be avoided by using vacuum collection (**B**). The *arrows* show movement of plunger during collection of cement

Table 2. Number, size, and volume of macropores and density using cement collection under vacuum (median, range). (Data from Wang et al. [13])

Pressure (bar)	Number of macropores cm^{-3}	Macropore diameter (mm)	Macropore volume (%)	Density (g cm^{-3})
0.2	0.2 (0.1–0.5)	1.50 (1.50–2.50)	0.04 (0.0–0.14)	1.283 (1.279–1.286)
0.05	0	0	0	1.287 (1.282–1.302)

Table 3. Porosity of bone cement using two vacuum levels, one at MMA boiling and one at no-boiling. (Data from Müller-Wille and Lidgren [16])

	Macropore area %		Micropores/ 63.8mm^{-2}		Density (g cm^{-3})		MMA volume (ml)	
(Bar)	0.12	0.01	0.12	0.01	0.12	0.01	0.12	0.01
Palacos® R	0.33	0.04	0.43	0.65	1.292	1.290	0	<0.1
SD	0.17	0.05	0.31	0.87	0.002	0.004		
	$p<0.001$		NS ($p=0.3$)		$p<0.01$			
Simplex® P	0.28	0.08	0.85	0.60	1.243	1.242	0	<0.1
SD	0.27	0.09	0.66	0.29	0.003	0.004		
	NS ($p=0.07$)		NS ($p=0.34$)		NS ($p=0.19$)			

of monomer boiling at room temperature (21°C). Müller-Wille and Lidgren [16] tested two cements, Palacos® R and Simplex P in Optivac® mixing system at 0.12 bar when no boiling of the MMA occurred and 0.01 bar which lead to MMA boiling. They measured the macropores, micropores, density, and amount of MMA lost during boiling. The higher vacuum (0.01 bar) almost completely eliminated macropores with no significant difference in micropores between boiling (0.01 bar) and no boiling (0.12 bar) of MMA (Table 3). Their explanation was that voids containing gaseous monomer collapse and the monomer gas condenses when the mixture is again subjected to atmospheric pressure. Therefore, increasing the vacuum level to the point of MMA "boiling" does not have an adverse effect on the porosity of the cement, but may even further reduce the porosity when combined with vacuum collection. A limited amount of monomer is evaporated during boiling, but this evaporation should not cause adverse effects for the cured cement. Caution must be used to avoid monomer leakage into the vacuum tube preventing higher vacuum.

Different Vacuum Mixing Systems

Vacuum mixing has been shown to remove micropores efficiently, but macropores (1–3 mm in diameter) still remain in the cement [1, 8, 13, 14, 17, 18]. Several systems have been developed and they have different characteristics. These differences include vacuum level, mixing method, mixing paddle and size of mixing container, all of which may influence the quality of cement.

Wang et al. [14] investigated several commercial vacuum mixing systems and cements. The mixing systems were Cemvac®, VCS®, Mitvac®, Optivac®, Osteobond®, and Stryker® (Fig. 3) and the cements Palacos® R and Simplex® P. The vacuum levels and the mixing methods are summarized in Table 4.

All vacuum mixing systems reduced micropores 10- to 100-fold and increased the density compared with open-bowl mixing. Reduction of number of macropores compared with open-bowl mixing was found in both Palacos® R and Simplex® P cement. Although all vacuum mixing systems reduced the

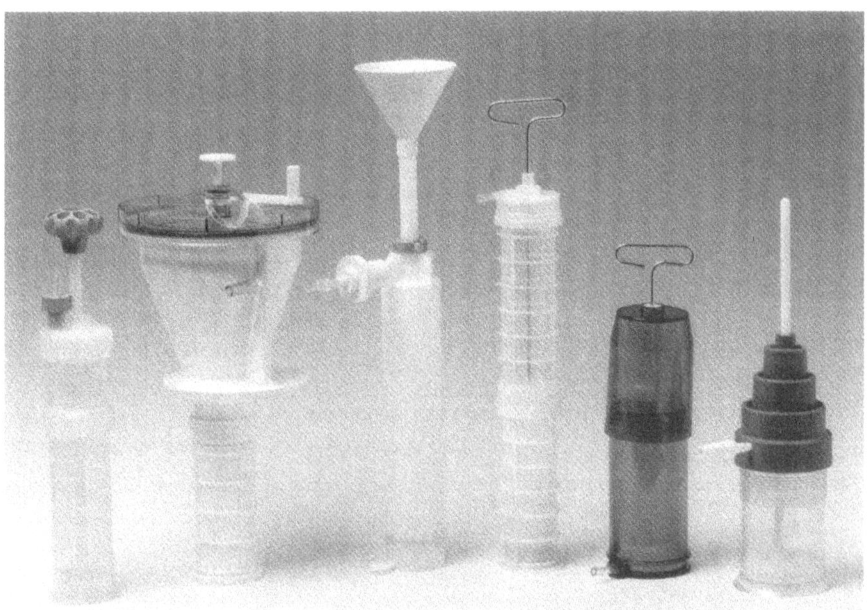

Fig. 3. The different vacuum mixing systems, picture from Wang et al. [14]. From *left to right*: Optivac®, Stryker®, Cemvac®, Osteobond®, Mitvac®, and VCS® systems

Table 4. Mixing methods and pressure levels in different vacuum mixing systems. (Data from Wang et al. [14])

System	Mixing method	Vacuum level (bar)	Vacuum collection
Cemvac®	Longitudinal and rotational	0.2	No
VCS®	Rotational	0.05	No
Mitvac®	Longitudinal and rotational	0.2	No
Osteobond®	Longitudinal and rotational	0.2	No
Optivac®	Longitudinal and rotational	0.1	Yes
Stryker®	Rotational	0.1	Partial
Open bowl	Rotational	1.0	No

number of macropores, the sizes of the macropores did not seem to be decreased to the same extent. The Cemvac® system seemed to be less efficient than the others. The Optivac® and Stryker® systems significantly decreased the pore area percentage of macropores compared to other systems (Tables 5, 6).

The investigation indicated that all vacuum mixing systems were effective in reducing the number of micropores and in increasing the density of the bone cement, but not all the systems were effective in eliminating macropores. The elimination of macropores may be associated with two factors in these systems, i.e., a high vacuum and cement collection under vacuum. Alkire et al. [7] tested at 0.60, 0.47, 0.34, and 0.07 bar for cement mixing. A vacuum level below 0.47 bar (lower vacuum = higher pressure) was inade-

Table 5. Comparison of porosity and density in Palacos® R with different mixing systems (Mean±SD). (Data from Wang et al. [14])

Mixing system	Number of macropores cm^{-3}	Pore area (%)	Micropores[a]	Density (g cm^{-3})
Cemvac®	1.0±0.5	3.0±1.5	6.0±2.9	1.263±0.013
VCS®	0.4±0.4	1.3±1.1	0.4±0.5	1.284±0.002
Mitvac®	0.7±0.2	2.4±1.4	1.0±1.7	1.266±0.025
Osteobond®	0.6±0.3	2.2±1.0	1.7±1.3	1.279±0.005
Optivac®	0.1±0.1	0.2±0.1	0.1±0.1	1.282±0.002
Stryker®	0.4±0.2	1.1±0.9	0.7±0.6	1.282±0.004
Open bowl	1.2±0.2	3.6±1.6	95±23	1.193±0.008
p Value[b]	<0.002	<0.001	<0.001	<0.005

[a] Number of pores per cross section (78.5 cm^2).
[b] Kruskal-Wallis test within the six vacuum mixing systems.

Table 6. Comparison of porosity and density in Simplex® P with different mixing systems (mean±SD). (Data from Wang et al. [14])

Mixing system	Number of macropores cm^{-3}	Pore area (%)	Micropores[a]	Density (g cm^{-3})
Osteobond®	0.4±0.3	1.3±0.7	3.4±4.4	1.232±0.015
Optivac®	0.1±0.1	0.1±0.2	0.7±0.6	1.240±0.003
Stryker®	0.1±0.1	0.3±0.2	0.8±0.5	1.241±0.001
Open bowl	1.8±0.2	4.8±1.1	90±48	1.176±0.020
p Value[b]	<0.02	<0.01	<0.05	<0.1

[a] Number of pores per cross section (78.5 cm^2).
[b] Kruskal-Wallis test within the three vacuum mixing systems.

quate for minimizing porosity. A nearly pore-free product could be achieved at 0.07 bar. The VCS® system using a 0.05-bar vacuum was more effective than Cemvac®, Osteobond®, and Mitvac® systems in decreasing macropores. Although the VCS® system reduced the number of macropores, the remaining macropores were still larger than with the Optivac® and Stryker® systems. This result may be due to air being re-entrapped in the cement when the vacuum is released and the cement collected. When collecting under vacuum as in the Optivac® system, air may not be as easily re-entrapped in the compacted cement [13]. The Mitvac® system is no longer marketed and the Cemvac® system has been changed.

A recent study from Wilkinson et al. [3] investigated the effect of mixing technique on the properties of bone cement. They used cylinder-type vacuum mixing systems (Optivac®, Cemvac®, and Summit®) with vacuums of 0.15, 0.2, and 0.25 bar and combined vacuum collection (such as in Optivac®) compared with bowl mixing system with vacuum (0.6 bar). The results showed the cylinder-mixed cement had fewer micropores and macropores, and also greater density, bending modulus, and bending strength than bowl-mixed cement. Once again the results proved that vacuum level and collection of the cement under vacuum is important in reducing porosity.

Different Cements

The vast majority of cements are based on the same chemical substance, i.e., methylmethacrylate (MMA), after mixing liquid and powder, the final material is polymethylmethacrylate (PMMA), but the properties of bone cement are not all alike. In addition to MMA, bone cements may contain other methacrylates, different radiopacifiers (zirconium dioxide or barium sulfate), different amounts of initiator and accelerator that initiate polymerization and control the setting time, different size and shape of powder particles that will influence the volume and viscosity, and contain different amounts or types of antibiotics. The different combinations will change the cement characteristics. It is not clear whether all cements will be free of pores when mixed in vacuum. We investigated the cement porosity of different cements that were mixed in the same brand of vacuum mixing system. The Optivac® system was chosen because it is one of the most efficient systems for porosity reduction of bone cement [3, 14, 15] and provides different sizes for different amount of cements (Fig. 4).

Palacos® R, Simplex® P, Palamed®, Osteopal®, and Osteobond® cements were used. The different packages of cement contained 40, 66, 80, and 120 g

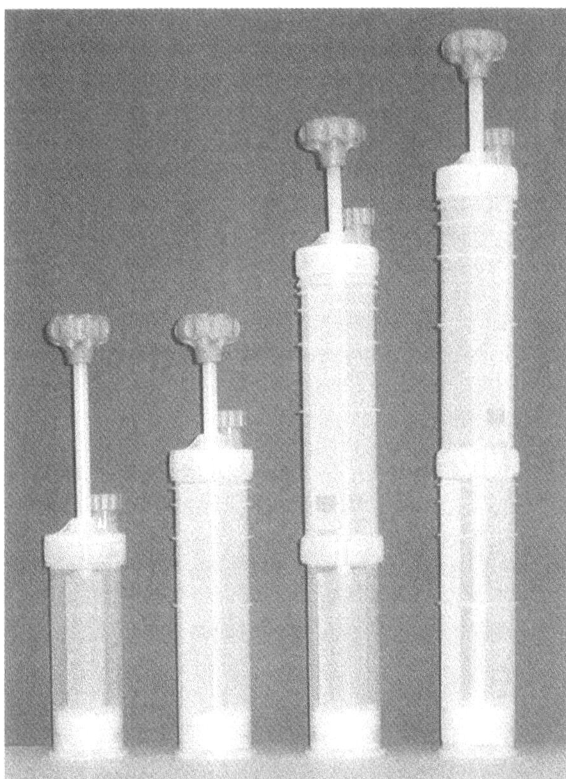

Fig. 4. Four sizes of Optivac® mixing systems are used for different amount of cement

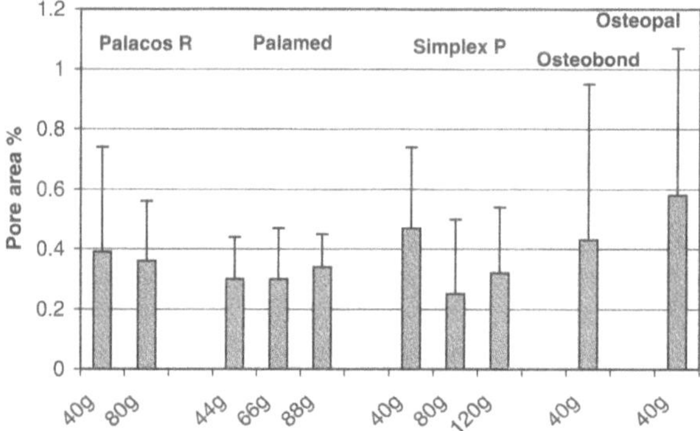

Fig. 5. The pore area (%) in different bone cements (mean±SD)

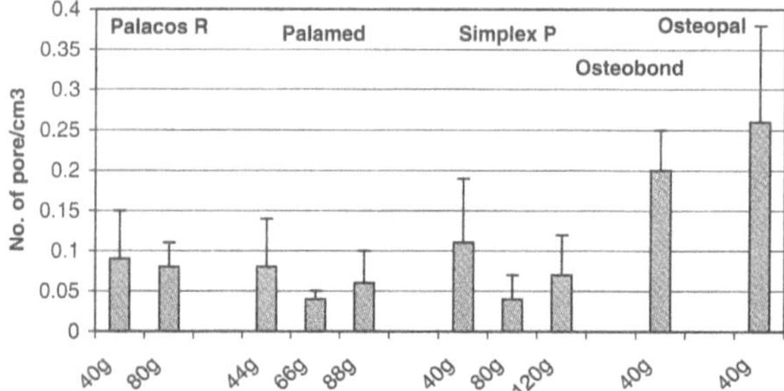

Fig. 6. Number of pores in different bone cements (mean±SD)

depending on the brand of cement. All the cements were mixed in the recommended size of Optivac® mixing system under a vacuum of 0.12 bar, according to specific mixing charts and instructions for each type of cement from the manufacturer of the mixing system.

The results showed that the pore areas were between 0.2% and 0.5% for all cements and amounts of cement (Fig. 5). The number of macropores was in the range of 0.04–0.26 pores per cm^3 for all specimens (Fig. 6). There were significant differences in the number of macropores in Palacos® R, Palamed®, and Simplex® P compared to Osteobond® and Osteopal®. The later cements produced more pores than the former, but the pore area showed no significant differences, indicating that the pores were relatively smaller than in the former. These different sizes of macropores from different bone cements may be caused by different viscosities (Table 7). Lower viscosity cement leads to more pores than higher viscosity cement. This corresponds to the physical property of viscosity, i.e., more small pores in low viscosity and fewer larger pores in high viscosity, when air is released through the different viscosity liquids (Fig. 7). This observation demonstrates that each bone cement can have its own optimal mixing technique.

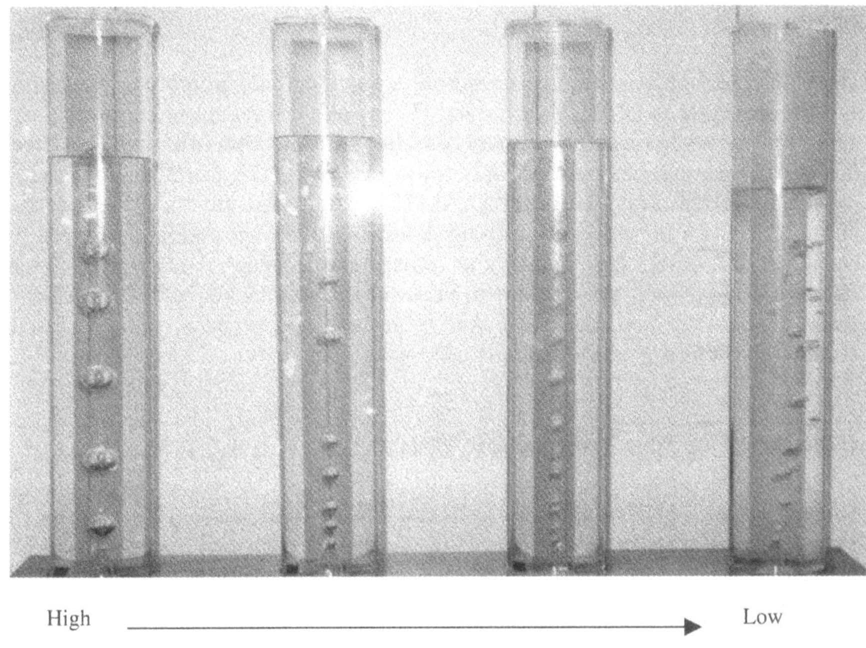

Fig. 7. Size and number of released air bubbles in liquids of different viscosity. High-to-low viscosity is *left to right*

Table 7. Bone cement viscosity. (Summarized by Kühn [12])

Bone cement	Manufacturer	Viscosity type
Palacos® R	Merck Biomaterial	High
Palacos® R	Schering Plough	High
Palamed®	Merck Biomaterial	High
Simplex® P	Howmedica	Medium
Osteobond®	Zimmer	Low
Osteopal®	Merck Biomaterial	Low

Mixing Speed

Some studies [19, 20] found a relationship between fast mixing and large pores and slow mixing and small pores for Simplex® P, Palacos® R, and Sulfix® mixed at atmospheric pressure. They also found that low viscosity cement needs a higher rate of mixing to get better cement quality. There is a shortage of information on mixing speed under vacuum. Most researchers recommend a rate of mixing of about 1 to 2 Hz [8, 15, 21, 22].

Stirrer

The materials of stirrers are commonly polyethylene, polypropylene, poly-tetrafluoroethylene (PTFE), and metal. There are several types of mixing stirrers, for example spatula, mixing paddle, mixing rod, and screw stirrer. These stirrers are for different methods of mixing, for example, horizontal, or rotational mixing. Draenert et al. [23] suggested that a PTFE-covered round stirring rod was advantageous because it does not adhere to bone cement. Kurdy et al. [24] found that rotating-axis system decrease porosity compared with fixed-axis system in vacuum mixing. In general, the design of stirrer should be considered so that monomer and powder can have better contact allowing for homogeneous mixing of cement.

Evacuation of Air from Powder Before Mixing

Schreurs et al. [21], Wang et al. [13] and Müller-Wille et al. [15] studied experimental vacuum-mixing set-ups that allowed the vacuum to be present before the powder and monomer were combined and vacuum was kept during the mixing, in order to evacuate air from powder (Fig. 8). They held the vacuum for 10 s after the maximal level had been reached and the monomer was added in powder. The devices yielded further reduction of porosity than commercial vacuum mixing systems. Therefore, it may be beneficial in reducing porosity to evacuate air from powder before mixing.

General Discussion

Although the literature on bone cement is voluminous, relatively few studies have reported the effect of vacuum mixing methods on the porosity of bone

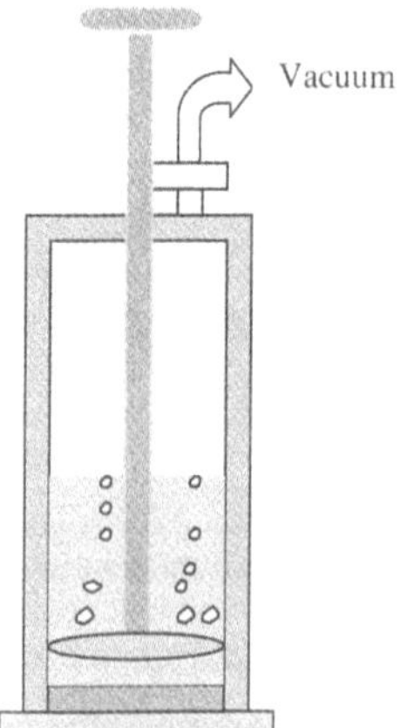

Fig. 8. Illustration of evacuation of air from bone cement powder

cement. This investigation may help orthopedic surgeons to know why and how a difference of cement porosity occurs when using vacuum mixing and why they should consider that different cements match a certain vacuum mixing system. Usually, the users have no idea of such combinations. If the cement, vacuum mixing system properties and mixing technique were not considered, the quality of various cements would be unknown. In recent clinical observations, we can see a trend. Earlier reports from the Swedish National Hip Registry suggested that for the first 4–5 years there was no significantly lower risk ratio [25] when vacuum was compared with manual mixing. However, in the latest reports [26, 27], the risk ratio decreased to 0.74. One reason for this may be improvements in the vacuum-mixing systems.

According to the studies of porosity in vacuum-mixing systems, we think that the pore area of cured bone cement should be less than 1%. An increase in macropores will increase the risk of fatigue failure. The current opinion is that efforts should be made to minimize the number and size of macropores.

Whether or not porosity reduction in acrylic bone cement is clinically relevant needs to be further investigated. In most studies the actual porosity has not been known or measured. Various experimental studies have shown that vacuum mixing of cement increases the cement longevity in fatigue testing [22, 23, 28]. However, clinical follow-up studies have not, as yet, been able to verify this result in situ. The incorrect use of vacuum mixing systems will decrease the cement quality and increase the variability of fatigue strength [29]. When investigating mixing systems, the porosity of the bone cement samples should always be stated in some way, for example, in standard tension tests; the data should also include the number and size of pores in used and discarded samples. This information will help readers to know the quality of cement produced by the mixing system.

This study also suggests that when manufacturers design new vacuum-mixing systems, they should always consider the quality of cement after mixing and provide instructions on how to mix different cements in their mixing systems to obtain optimal cement quality. It reminds users to investigate what cement quality they will get and the necessity to use a mixing system correctly.

In conclusion, factors within a vacuum mixing system that may reduce the formation of porosity are: the use of high vacuum, optimal stirrer, controlled mixing speed, the prevention of air entrapment during cement collection, and the use of matched mixing system for special cement viscosity and cement volume. Future vacuum mixing systems may benefit from evacuation of air from the powder before mixing. When an optimal combination of cement and mixing system is used, cement quality can be assured.

Acknowledgements. This study was supported by the Swedish Medical Research Council (project 09509). The authors wish to thank Professor K.E. Tanner for her critical reading of the manuscript and Dr. Ernst Jonsson for introducing us to vacuum mixing.

References

1. Lidgren L, Drar H, Möller J (1984) Strength of polymethylmethacrylate increased by vacuum mixing. Acta Orthop Scand 55:536–541
2. Lewis G. Nyman J, Trieu HH (1997a) Effect of mixing method on selected properties of acrylic bone cement. J Biomed Mater Res 38:221–228
3. Wilkinson, JM, Eveleigh R, Hamer AJ, Milne A, Miles AW, Stockley I (2000) Effect of mixing technique on the properties of acrylic bone-cement. A comparison of syringe and bowl mixing systems. J Arthroplasty 15:663–667
4. Carter DR, Gates EI, Harris WH (1982) Strain-controlled fatigue of acrylic bone cement. J Biomed Mater Res 24:135–154
5. James, SP, Jasty M, Davies J, Piehler A (1992) A fractographic investigation of PMMA bone cement focusing on the relationship between porosity reduction and increased fatigue life. J Biomed Mater Res 26:651–662
6. Topoleski, LDT, Ducheyne P, Cuckler JM (1990) A fractographic analysis of *in vivo* poly (methylmethacrylate) bone cement failure mechanisms. J Biomed Mater Res 245:135–154
7. Alkire MJ, Dabezies EJ, Hastings PR (1987) High vacuum as a method of reducing porosity of polymethylmethacrylate. Orthopedics 10:1533–1539
8. Wixson RL, Lautenschlager EP, Novak MA (1987) Vacuum mixing of acrylic bone cement. J Arthroplasty 2:141–149
9. Bishop N E, Ferguson S, Tepic S (1996) Porosity reduction in bone cement at the cement-stem interface. J Bone Joint Surg [Br] 78-B:349–356.
10. Wang JS, Flivik G, Taylor M, Lidgren L (1999) Stem-cement interface shear strength is influenced by stem surface finish but not cement interface porosity. 45th ORS, Anaheim, Calif., USA
11. Wang JS, Goodman SB, Franzén H, Aspenberg P, Lidgren L (1993) The effect of vacuum mixing on the microscopic homogenicity of Palacos R bone cement. Eur J Exp Musculoskel Res 2:159–165
12. Kühn KD (2000) Bone Cement. Springer, Berlin Heidelberg New York
13. Wang JS, Franzén H, Jonsson E, Lidgren L (1993) Porosity of bone cement reduced by mixing and collecting under vacuum. Acta Orthop Scand 64:143–146
14. Wang JS, Toksvig-Larsen S, Müller-Wille P, Franzén H (1996) Is there any difference between vacuum mixing systems in reducing bone cement porosity? J Biomed Mater Res (Applied Biomater) 33:115–119
15. Müller-Wille P, Wang JS, Lidgren L (1997) Integrated system for preparation of bone cement and effects on cement quality and environment. J Biomed Mater Res (Applied Biomater) 38:135–142
16. Müller-Wille P, Lidgren L (1996) Boiling of monomer during high vacuum mixing of bone cement does not increase cement porosity. 6th EORS Conference, Bergen Norway, pp 50
17. Linden U, Gillquist J (1989) Air inclusion in bone cement. Importance of the mixing technique. Clin Othop 247:148–151
18. Davies JP, Harris WH (1990) Optimization and comparison of three vacuum mixing systems of porosity reduction of Simplex P cement. Clin Orthop 254:261–269
19. Lee AJC (1984) The effect of mixing technique and surgical technique on the properties of bone cement. Presented at the Knochenzement Symposium, March 23–25
20. Eyerer P, Jin R (1986) Influence of mixing technique on some properties of PMMA bone cement. J Biomed Mater Res 20:1057–1094
21. Schreurs BW, Spierings PTJ, Husikes R, Slooff TJJH (1988) Effects of preparation techniques on the porosity of acrylic cements. Acta Orthop Scand 59:403–409
22. Lewis G (1997b) Properties of acrylic bone cement: state of the art review. J Biomed Mater Res (Appl Biomater) 38:155–182
23. Draenert K, Draenert Y, Garde U Ulrich CH (1999) Manual of cementing technique. Springer, Berlin Heidelberg New York
24. Kurdy NMG, Hodgkinson JP, Haynes R (1996) Acrylic bone-cement. Influence of mixer design and unmixed powder. J Arthroplasty 11:813–819
25. Malchau H, Herberts Peter (1998) Prognosis of total hip replacement. 65th Annual Meeting of the American Academy of Orthopedic Surgeons, USA
26. Malchau H, Herberts P (2000) Prognosis of total hip replacement. 67th Annual Meeting of the American Academy of Orthopedic Surgeons, USA
27. Söderman P (2000) On the validity of the results from the Swedish National Total Hip Arthroplasty Register Acta Orthop Scand Suppl 296:1–71

28. Harper EJ, Bonfield W (2000) Tensile characteristics of ten commercial acrylic bone cements. J Biomed Mater Res 53:605–616
29. Murphy BP, Prendergast PJ (2000) Quantification of the variability in fatigue life of PMMA bone cement in relation to mixing technique. 46th Annual Meeting of Orthopedics Research Society, March, Orlando, Florida, USA, pp 252

Efficacy of a New Prepacked Vacuum Mixing System with Palamed® G Bone Cement

KATRIN SCHELLING, STEFFEN J. BREUSCH

Abstract. We determined macro-, micro- and total porosity and bending strength (ISO 5833) of prechilled Palacos® R mixed under vacuum by using Optivac® systems and Palamed® G mixed both with Optivac® and GZS® mixing systems. All cement specimens that we tested fulfilled the ISO requirements. The lowest total porosity and macroporosity scores (for extruded cement) were obtained with the combination Palamed® G/Optivac®. The lowest microporosity (<1 mm) was determined for Palacos® R/Optivac®, but no statistical significance was recorded between the groups/combinations. Our results confirm the high efficacy of both mixing systems. Palamed® G bone cement, which does not require prechilling, yielded marginally better mechanical properties and lower porosities (with Optivac®) than Palacos® R but controlled clinical studies are essential before widespread use.

Introduction

Aseptic loosening continues to be the most common cause of failure [30, 31] following cemented total hip arthroplasty (THA). There is little doubt that the use of modern cementing techniques in THA reduces the risk for revision [30, 31] and results in improved long-term outcome [5, 7, 34, 38, 39, 42], even in young patients [3, 4, 35]. Modern cementing techniques aim to improve the interlock between bone and cement and thus to establish a durable interface [20]. Failure and loosening of a cemented implant may occur at this biological interface but can also originate from the interface between cement and implant [10, 33] and within the cement mantle [20, 42, 44] itself. Thin but complete cement layers on compact bone can resist deformation for many years without fracturing [11]. However, a thin layer of cement has less potential for energy absorption and is more vulnerable to crack and fail [44]. Fractures or even complete ruptures of the cement mantle are well recognized [11, 12, 20] and can be associated with the use of distal centralizers [6]. Local defects in the cement mantle have also been reported with large straight "cemented press-fit" stems, especially vadjacent to sharp corners of the implant [12]. Osteolysis and granuloma formation [2, 36] may occur as a consequence in close relationship to complete fractures within the cement mantle. Such fractures are also commonly observed in vitro [23, 37] and in vivo [20, 44] in the presence of large voids and flaws within the cement, which may lead to a rapid propagation of cement cracks [8, 19]. Macroporosity has been shown to correlate with reduced fatigue strength and mechanical failure [15, 19]. Reduction of cement porosity is a logical step in the attempt to improve the quality and fatigue life of cement. Vacuum mixing has been shown to be effective in achieving these objectives in vitro [1, 21, 23, 26, 27, 47], in particular in achieving reduction of microporosity [27, 46, 47]. A satisfactory reduction of macroporosity, however, may not be achieved with vacuum mixing, unless not only mixing but also collection of the cement is done under vacuum [45]. Wang et al. [46] have demonstrated that not all vacuum systems are equally effective in reducing the number and size of large voids. A high efficacy in this context can be achieved by combining Palacos® R cement and Optivac® mixing systems [46]. The recent results from the Swedish national hip registry [31] have proven that both the use of Palacos® R and vacuum mixing reduce the revision risk for loosening. However, Palacos® R has the disadvantage of requiring prechilling [11, 17, 41, 45] for porosity reduction and successful evacuation of entrapped air. Thus, great discipline and motivation in maintaining adequate storage and mixing conditions are mandatory. Based on the long-term clinical success of Palacos® R a new bone cement Palamed® G and a new mixing system (GZS®) have been developed in an attempt to provide simplification and improved handling characteristics.

The aim of this study was to investigate the properties of this new cement and the efficacy of the new mixing system in reducing the macro- and microporosity when compared with Palacos® R and Optivac® as a gold standard.

Materials and Methods

Specimen Preparation

All mixing procedures were performed by the same investigator (K.S.), who had been instructed by the manufacturers to ensure correct handling of the systems. Three mixes with each system/combination were performed to account for the learning curve. For evaluation 10 samples with Palacos® R/ Optivac®, Palamed® G/Optivac® and Palamed® G/GZS® were produced under identical, standardized laboratory conditions at 19 °C room temperature. Vacuum levels and mixing protocols given by the manufacturers were strictly implemented.

Palacos® R (Ch.221196, identical batch: 2791, Biomet-Merck) was prechilled to 4 °C and mixed under vacuum using Optivac® mixing systems (Mebio, Scandimed). Two packages (81.6 g polymer powder, 40 ml monomer liquid) were used for preparation of the test specimens. The powder was added to the monomer placed in the mixing cartridge; after a waiting phase of 10 s to allow for build up of a vacuum, the mixing process was commenced. After stirring for 30 s and collection of the cement at the top of the cartridge the vacuum was disconnected and the nozzle securely locked.

The cement was extruded from the cement gun at 2 min and 30 s after mixing into 15 ml plastic tubes (Greiner, Heidelberg) in a retrograde manner to simulate operative conditions. With the same mix a thin plate of cement ($100 \times 80 \times 3.3$ mm) was produced by injecting cement into a teflon-coated metal mold (Tetrafluorethylentelomer PTFE Klingerflon® Spray, Klinger GmbH, Idstein-Taunus). The remaining cement was left to cure in the nozzle. The cement specimens for porosity determination were obtained by breaking off the plastic.

The same protocol was used for Palamed®G/GZS® and Palamed® G/Optivac® (Palamed® G = Gentamicin, batch: Ch.100299, Kulzer). With Optivac® the identical steps were followed as with the use of Palacos® R. GZS® is a prepacked system containing 61.2 g polymer powder to be mixed with 30 ml monomer. A cartridge with the monomer is screwed below the polymer prepacked cartridge thus allowing the powder to fall into the liquid.

Standardised radiographs (35 kV, 4 mAs, 60 cm film-focus distance [FFD]) of the cement cylinders from the nozzles and the plastic tubes were taken with a Faxitron (Modell 43855 C, Rohde & Schwarz, Köln) using high resolution mammography films (Microvision C, mammography film, 18×24 cm, Sterling Diagnostic Imaging, USA).

Further preparation was done using a diamond circular saw (Grünewald PSI Medizintechnik) with water cooling to prevent overheating. Four 5 mm slices were obtained from both cylinders and nozzles. From the nozzles 2 cement slices were taken from the proximal and distal ends, respectively. From the cylinders 4 consecutive slices from the proximal end were used for analysis. Microradiographs were taken (25 kV, 4 mAs, 60 cm FFD) from all cement slices.

The cement plates for mechanical testing were cut to strips with smaller dimensions ($80 \times 10 \times 3.3$ mm) and were placed in a water bath at $37\,^{\circ}$C for 48 h following 14 days storage at room temperature – as required by ISO 5833.

Test Protocol

Porosity

The test protocol involved porosity measurements and mechanical testing according to ISO 5833 (4-point bending test).

Macroporosity ($\geq$1 mm)

The largest pore diameter was measured and recorded by using the radiographs of the cement cylinders. Categories of 1–2 mm (C1), 3–5 mm (C2) and >5 mm (C3) were defined. A macroporosity score was calculated by multiplying C1 by 2.25, C2 by 16 and C3 by 36. The factors for multiplication were received by squaring the mean pore sizes of each category, (i.e. 1.5, 4, 6). For each sample a total score was thus obtained.

Total Porosity

All microradiographs were digitized by using a scanner and analyzed by using an image analysis software (Kontron KS 300, Kontron Elektronik GmbH, Carl Zeiss Vision). Total porosity was recorded as a percentage per total cement area.

Microporosity (<1 mm)

To record all micropores that were not detectable radiographically a microscopic surface analysis was performed. The surfaces of one slice per cylinder were prepared by using grinding paper (800) and black shoe polish to stain all surface irregularities/grooves representing pores. The remaining polish was removed from the cement surface by using a razor blade. A light microscope (SZ6045TR, Olympus, Japan) with two light sources (Highlight 3000 Type 8550 N, Olympus, Hamburg) was used and all images were digitized with 1.5-fold magnification by using a digital camera (3CCD Color Video Camera DXC-950P, Sony, Japan).

Mechanical Testing

Bending strength was tested according to ISO 5833. The standardized narrow cement strips were removed from the water bath (see above) and placed on the testing device. A compression device (Universalprüfmaschine Frank 81816/B No. 28742) with a maximal load of 100 N and a constant speed of 5 mm/min was used until fracture of the specimens occurred. In cases where no fracture took place the maximal load was recorded before the specimens underwent plastic deformation.

Statistical Analysis

For statistical analysis a Scheffé test was used for comparison of macroporosity, total porosity, microporosity and bending strength. Differences with a P-value equal to or less than 0.05 were considered significant.

Results

All specimens showed a homogenous distribution of the radiopaque agent with no apparent macroscopic, microscopic or radiographic irregularities.

Macroporosity (≥1 mm)

The combination Palamed® G/Optivac® showed the lowest macroporosity scores in the extruded cylinder specimens. There was no significant difference between the other two groups (cylinders) and no difference between the three groups for the nozzle specimens. Macroporosity was greater in the (extruded) cylinders (Fig. 1) than in the specimens obtained from the nozzles (Fig. 2), but larger pores were recorded in the nozzles.

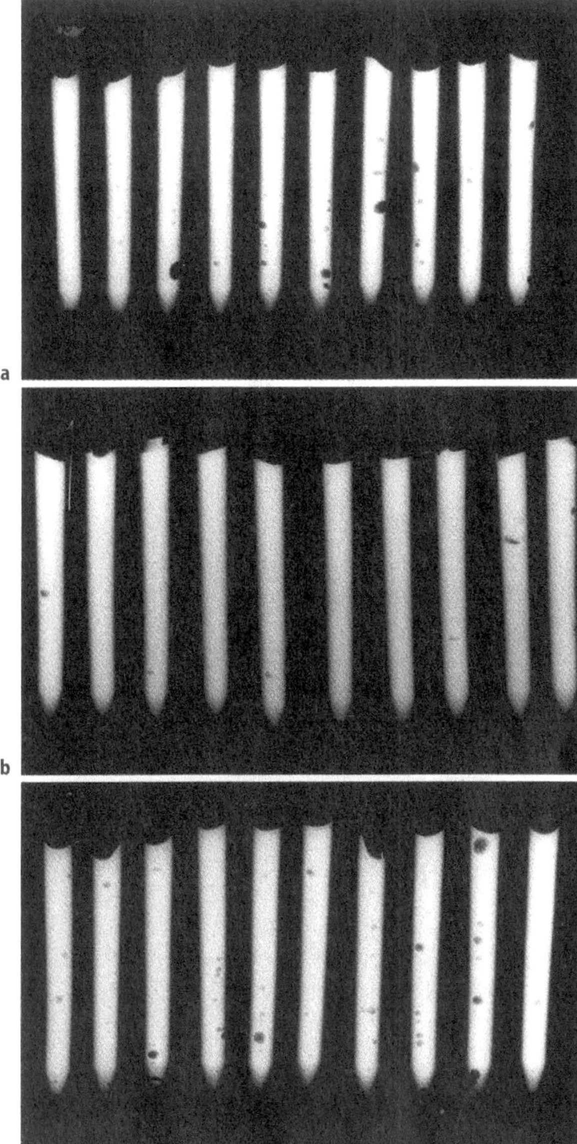

Fig. 1 a–c. Microradiographs of extruded cement. Note: No significant differences were found between macroporosity scores.
a Palamed® G/GZS®;
b Palamed® G/Optivac®;
c Palacos® R/Optivac®

Total Porosity

The combination Palamed® G/Optivac® yielded the lowest total porosity (0.8±0.9%) in the cylinder specimens. The mean total porosity was 11.7±7.8% for Palamed® G/GZS® and 3.7±2.2% for Palacos® R/Optivac® for the slices from the extruded cement. The highest porosity was recorded for nozzle specimens obtained from Palamed® G/Optivac®. The mean total porosity from the nozzle specimens showed no difference between the remaining

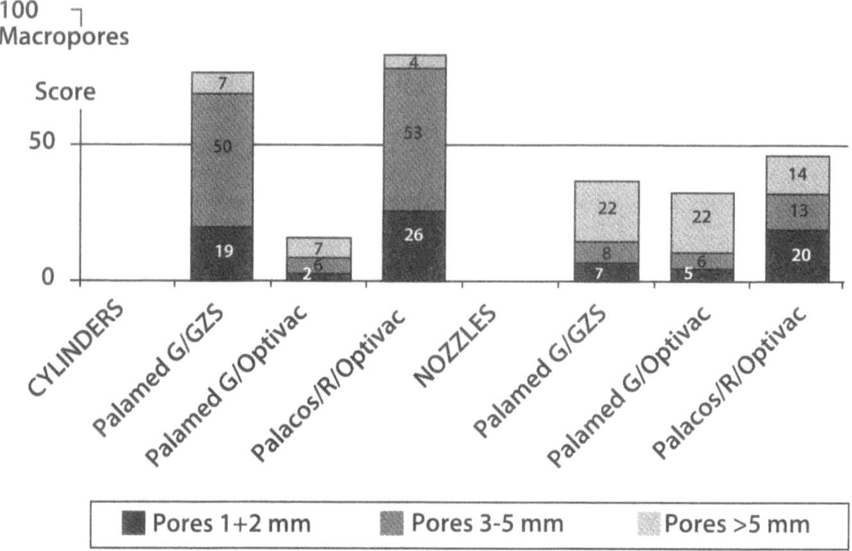

Fig. 2. Macroporosity scores

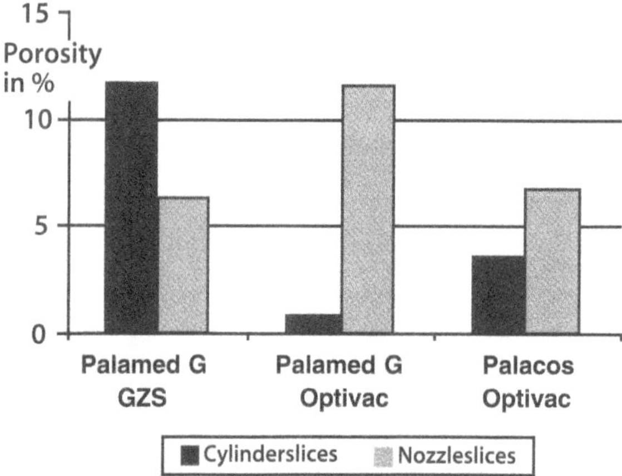

Fig. 3. Total porosity

groups: 6.4±8.7% for Palamed® G/GZS® and 6.9±18.7% for Palacos® R/Optivac®, respectively (Fig. 3).

Microporosity (<1 mm)

The microscopic determination of microporosity (Fig. 4) revealed no significant difference between Palamed® G/Optivac® (1.13±0.18%) and Palamed® G/GZS® (1.43±0.34%), but a difference when compared with Palacos® R/Optivac® (0.48±0.35%).

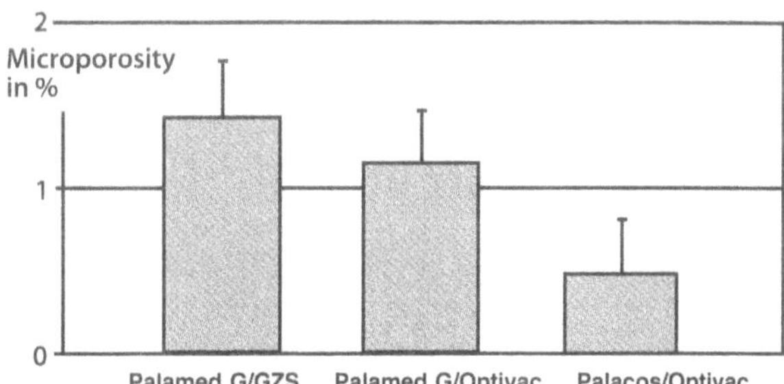

Fig. 4. Microporosity

Bending Strength

All test specimens fulfilled the requirements, according to the international standards, with a minimal bending strength of 50 MPa (ISO 5833). The mean bending strength (to fracture) was 59.7±1.5 MPa for Palamed® G/GZS® and 63.9±4.4 MPa for Palamed® G/Optivac® (Fig. 5). None of the Palacos® R specimens fractured and the maximal load was recorded for comparison at 56.2 ±3.6 MPa before plastic deformation occurred (Fig. 6). Using these maximal values only significant differences between Palamed® G/Optivac® and Palacos® R/Optivac® were observed ($P<0.05$).

Discussion

Pores within the cement can arise from air contained and trapped within the polymer powder, air introduced during stirring (mixing process) or during transfer of the mixture into a non-vented cement gun and monomer boiling during polymerization [47]. All the systems/combinations investigated eliminate air by the simple mechanism that air entrapped within the polymer powder is extracted under vacuum and remaining air can escape when the polymer beads fall into the monomer liquid. Also, both mixing systems allow for collection of the cement under vacuum [45] and no tilting or cement transfer into a delivery gun is necessary.

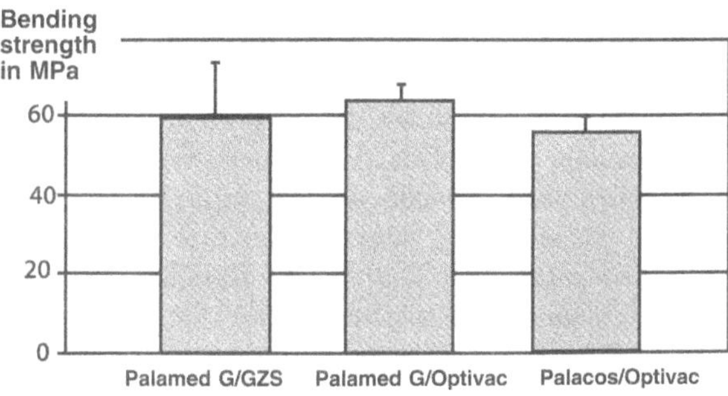

Fig. 5. Bending strength
(ISO 5833)

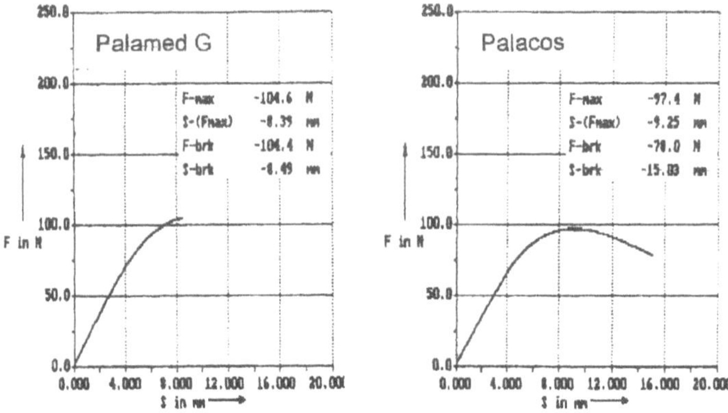

Fig. 6. Bending curves for Palamed® G and Palacos® R

Davies and Harris [9] showed in their study that larger cement mixes were less susceptible to inhomogeneity than smaller mixes (80 g compared with 40 g). In our study no apparent difference was observed in this respect although the GZS® only accommodates 60 g polymer. Draenert [11] emphasized that the size of the mixing cartridge/bowl needs to be adapted to the cement volume.

The similar macroporosity scores of all three groups in the specimens taken from the nozzles indicate similar efficacy of the mixing systems investigated. It is of note that in the nozzle specimens of all three groups there was a substantial percentage of pores larger than 5 mm. This may due to entrapped air not entirely evacuated or due to monomer void formation during polymerization with significant temperature peaks, but these speculations must remain assumptions. Meyer et al. [32] demonstrated void formation and increased porosity secondary to monomer "boiling" in cement layers thicker than 8 mm. No in vivo experiments exist to our knowledge that could provide more information to explain the mechanism of large void formation. However, this finding is of doubtful clinical significance as this portion of cement (in the nozzle) is usually discarded.

In contrast, Palamed® G/Optivac® provided the lowest macroporosity scores in the extruded cement specimens. This is probably the porosity that matters most in the clinical context [15, 19, 43], as this phenomenon can be responsible for large void formation. Large voids are more prone to crack initiation than smaller pore sizes [19]. Interestingly, only for Palamed® G/ Optivac® the macroporosity decreased with cement extrusion. The other two combinations yielded far higher porosity scores after cement application with predominant pore sizes of 3–5 mm. One possible cause is the difference in cement volume between nozzles (approximately 7.5–8 ml) and extruded cylinders (15 ml). This would mean that in proportion the macroporosities in extruded and nozzle cement are comparable. However, this does not explain why for Palamed® G/Optivac® more large voids were recorded in the nozzle. The most satisfactory explanation for this discrepancy is the hypothesis that large voids adjacent to the inner wall of the nozzle do not intermix with the cement during extrusion – if the voids do not emerge in the nozzle during polymerization after cement extrusion. Whether the eccentricity of the nozzle attachment to the mixing cartridge in the Optivac® system plays an important role for this finding remains unknown.

Wang et al. [27] also examined both nozzles and extruded cylinders but did not distinguish between these in their report. Also no account was given as to whether the cement samples were all mixed by the same investigator, although other studies have demonstrated the influence of the user upon mixing results [14, 16, 28]. As for macroporosity also for total porosity, Palamed® G/Optivac® yielded the best outcome but only in (the more important) extruded cement samples. The ideal overall porosity of bone cement remains unknown. Hahn et al. [16] showed that a further porosity reduction beyond 3–5% does not result in further improvement of stability.

Our results are in agreement with Wang et al. [46] who found the lowest macroporosity when Optivac® mixing systems were used. We can confirm the high efficacy of this mixing system. It is difficult to compare our findings with other reports from the literature as no standardized evaluation protocol has been accepted and too many other variables (temperature, humidity, time of cement extrusion, mixing protocol) play a role [1, 9, 13, 14, 41].

The designers of Palamed® set out to produce a bone cement with simple storing and handling characteristics. With regard to macroporosity this new cement showed an apparently better performance (without statistical significance) than Palacos® R when Optivac® systems were used.

However, with regard to microporosity reduction all combinations were highly efficient and the results compare with other reports [21, 41, 45, 46]. The lowest microporosity was recorded for Palacos® R, but the clinical relevance of reduction of microporosity remains subject to debate [25, 29, 37].

All cement specimens fulfilled the ISO bending strength requirements. The mechanical in vitro performance of Palamed® G appears at least equal to Palacos® R and was even superior in our experiment. It has been shown that reduced mechanical properties occur in some bone cements loaded with antibiotics, although with marginal effect [22, 24, 40]. The difference between Palamed® G and Palacos® R may have been more pronounced if Refobacin Palacos® R had been used. We could not find any reports in the literature that could support our finding that the Palacos® R strips did not fracture at the highest point of the bending curve, although the test requirements according to ISO 5833 were strictly followed. However, the clinical relevance of ISO 5833 has to be questioned as only static testing of material properties is implemented [18]. In the clinical situation bone cement is loaded dynamically and undergoes continuous creep deformation.

In conclusion, we found Palamed® G to be equal to Palacos® R with regard to porosity and bending strength, particularly when Optivac® systems are used. Nevertheless, controlled clinical trials and a careful "staged introduction" of this new cement are to be recommended before widespread clinical use.

References

1. Alkire MJ, Dabezies EJ, Hastings PR (1987) High vacuum as a method of reducing porosity of polymethylmethacrylate. Orthopedics 10:1533–1539
2. Anthony PP, Gie GA, Howie CR, Ling RSM (1990) Localised endosteal bone lysis in relation to the femoral components of cemented total hip arthroplasties. J Bone Joint Surg 72B:971–979
3. Ballard WT, Callaghan JJ, Sullivan PM, Johnston RC (1994) The results of improved cementing techniques for total hip arthroplasty in patients less than fifty years old. J Bone Joint Surg 76 A:959
4. Barrack RL, Mulroy RD, Harris WH (1992) Improved cementing techniques and femoral component loosening in young patients with hip arthroplasty. J Bone Joint Surg 74B:385
5. Beckenbaugh RD, Ilstrup DM (1978) Total hip arthroplasty. A review of three hundred and thirty-three cases with long follow-up. J Bone Joint Surg 60 A:306
6. Breusch SJ, Ewerbeck V, Lukoschek M (1999) Einflußfaktoren auf die Langlebigkeit des zementierten Hüftendoprothesenschaftes. Aktuelle Traumatologie 29:1–11
7. Britton AR, Murray DW, Bulstrode CJ, McPherson K, Denham RA (1996) Long-term comparison of Charnley and Stanmore design total hip replacements. J Bone Joint Surg 78B:802
8. Carter DR, Gates EI, Harris WH (1982) Strain-controlled fatigue of acrylic bone cement. Biomed Materials Res 16:647–657
9. Davies JP, Harris WH (1990) Optimization and comparison of three vacuum mixing systems for porosity reduction of Simplex. Clin Orthop Rel Res 254:261–269
10. Dowd JE, Cha CW, Trakru S, Kim SY, Yang IH, Rubash HE (1998) Failure of total hip arthroplasty with a precoated prosthesis. 4- to 11-year results. Clin Orthop 355:123–136
11. Draenert K (1998) Zur Praxis der Zementverankerung. In: Forschung und Fortbildung in der Chirurgie des Bewegungsapparates 2. München: Art and Science, pp 27–28
12. Draenert K, Draenert Y (1992). Die Adaptation des Knochens an die Deformation durch Implantate. Strain-Adaptive Bone Remodelling. In: Forschung und Fortbildung in der Chirurgie des Bewegungsapparates 3. München: Art and Science, S 42
13. Ege W (1984) Normung von Knochenzementen. In: Burri C, Harder F, Bauer R (eds): Aktuelle Probleme in Chirurgie und Orthopädie. Band 31 Knochenzement Willert HG, Buchhorn G (eds), Verlag Hans Huber, Bern Stuttgart Tokyo, pp 133–135
14. Eyerer P, Jin R (1986) Influence of mixing technique on some properties of PMMA bone cement. J Biomed Mater Res 20:1057–1094
15. Gilbert JL, Menis DW, Smith SM, Lautenschlager EP, Wixson RW (1990) Effect of pore size and morphology on fatigue crack initiation in acrylic bone cements. 16th Annual Meeting Society Biomaterials, Charleston SC, Trans 103
16. Hahn M, Engelbrecht E, Delling G (1990) Eine quantitative Analyse zur Bestimmung der Porosität von vorkomprimiertem und unter Vakuum gemischtem Knochenzement. Chirurg 61:512–517
17. Hansen D, Jensen JS (1990) Prechilling and vacuum mixing not suitable for all bone cements. Handling characteristics and exotherms of bone cements. J Arthroplasty 5: 287–290
18. Hansen D, Jensen JS (1992) Mixing does not improve mechanical properties of all bone cements. Acta Orthop Scand 63:13–18
19. James SP, Jasty M, Davies J, Piehler H (1992) A fractographic investigation of PMMA bone cement focusing on the relationship between porosity reduction and increased fatigue life. J Biomed Mater Res 26:651–662
20. Jasty M, Maloney WJ, Bragdon CR, O'Connor DO, Haire T, Harris WH (1991) The initiation of failure in cemented femoral components of hip arthroplasties. J Bone Joint Surg 73B:551–558
21. Kindt-Larsen T, Smith DB, Jensen JS (1995) Innovations in acrylic bone cement and application equipment. J Appl Biomat 6:75–83
22. Kühn KD (2000) Comparative tests of antibiotic-loaded cements. Bone cements. Up-to-date comparison of physical and chemical properties of commercial materials. Springer, Berlin Heidelberg New York, p 228
23. Kurdy NMG, Hodgkinson JP, Haynes R (1996) Acrylic bone-cement. Influence of mixer design and unmixed powder. J Arthroplasty 11:813–819
24. Lee AJC, Ling RS, Vangal SS (1978) Some clinically relevant variables affecting the mechanical behaviour of bone cement. Arch Orthop Traumat Surg 92:1–18
25. Lewis G, Nyman J, Trieu H (1998) The apparent fracture toughness of acrylic bone cement: effect of three variables. Biomaterials 19:961–967

26. Lidgren U, Drar H, Möller J (1984) Strength of polymethylmethacrylate increased by vacuum mixing. Acta Orthop Scand 55:536–541
27. Lidgren U, Bodelind B, Möller J (1987) Bone cement improved by vacuum mixing and chilling. Acta Orthop Scand 57:27–32
28. Linden U (1988) Porosity in manually mixed bone cement. Clin Orthop Rel Res 231:110–112
29. Ling RSM (1998) Porosity reduction in cement is not necessary for cemented total hip arthroplasty. The Hip Society and AAHKS, New Orleans
30. Malchau H, Herberts P (1998) Prognosis of total hip replacement in Sweden: Revision and re-revision rate in THR. Presented at the 65th Annual Meeting of the American Academy of Orthopaedic Surgeons, New Orleans
31. Malchau H, Herberts P, Söderman P, Odén A (2000) Prognosis of total hip replacement: Update and validation of results from the Swedish National Hip Arthroplasty Registry. 67th Annual Meeting of the American Academy of Orthopaedic Surgeons, Orlando, USA
32. Meyer PJ. Lautenschlager EP, Moore BK (1973) On the setting properties of acrylic bone cement. J Bone Joint Surg 55 A:149
33. Mohler CG, Callaghan JJ, Collis DK, Johnston RC (1995) Early loosening of the femoral component at the cement-prosthesis interface after total hip replacement. J Bone Joint Surg 77 A:1315–1322
34. Mulroy RD, Harris WH (1990) The effect of improved cementing techniques on component loosening in total hip replacement. An 11-year radiographic review. J Bone Joint Surg 72B:757
35. Mulroy RD, Harris WH (1997) Acetabular and femoral fixation 15 years after cemented total hip surgery. Clin Orthop 337:118
36. Pazzaglia UE (1990) Pathology of the bone-cement interface in loosening of total hip replacement. Arch Orthop Trauma Surg 109:83–88
37. Rimnac M, Wright TM, McGill D (1986) The effect of centrifugation on the fracture properties of acrylic bone cements. J Bone Joint Surg 68:281
38. Roberts DW, Poss R, Kelley K (1986) Radiographic comparison of cementing techniques in total hip arthroplasty. J Arthroplasty 1(4):241–247
39. Russotti GM, Coventry MB, Stauffer RN (1988) Cemented total hip arthroplasty with contemporary techniques. A five-year follow-up study. Clin Orthop 235:141
40. Schurman DJ, Swenson LW, Piziali RL (1978) Bone cement with and without antibiotics: A study of mechanical properties. In: The hip. Proceedings of the 6th Open Scientific Meeting of the Hip Society. CV Mosby, St.Louis, pp 87–96
41. Smeds S, Goertzen D, Ivarsson I (1997) Influence of temperature and vacuum mixing on bone cement properties. Clin Orthop Rel Res 334:326–334
42. Stauffer RN (1982) Ten year follow-up study of total hip replacement: with particular reference to roentgenographic loosening of the components. J Bone Joint Surg 64 A:983
43. Topoleski LDT, Ducheyne P, Cuckler JM (1995) The effects of centrifugation and titanium fiber reinforcement on fatigue failure mechanisms in polymethylmethacrylate bone cement. J Biomed Mater Res 29:299–307
44. Walde H-J, Rudigier J, Wagner R (1987) Beanspruchungsbedingte Strukturveränderungen des Knochenzementes – Untersuchungen an reoperierten Präparaten. In: Willert H-G, Buchhorn G (eds) Aktuelle probleme in Chirurgie und Orthopädie. Band 31, Hans Huber, Bern Stuttgart Toronto
45. Wang JS, Franzen H, Jonsson E, Lidgren L (1993) Porosity of bone cement reduced by mixing and collecting under vacuum. Acta Orthop Scand 64:143–146
46. Wang JS, Toksvig-Larsen S, Müller-Wille, Franzen H (1996) Is there any difference between vacuum mixing systems in reducing bone cement porosity? J Biomed Mater Res 33:115–119
47. Wixson RL, Lautenschlager EP, Novak MA (1987) Vacuum mixing of acrylic bone cement. J Arthroplasty 2(2):141–149

The Use of the Kent Hip in Fractures

Treatment of Periprospective Hip Fractures

A. L. RUIZ, J. G. BROWN

Abstract. Intraoperative and postoperative periprosthetic fractures can pose a difficult problem, and various surgical treatment options are available. We present our experience with the Kent hip in 33 patients. Surgical technique, peroperative details and complications are discussed. The combination of a hip prosthesis and intramedullary device provides the Kent hip with the necessary flexibility to deal with these complex fractures and is recommended as a good salvage procedure for an often elderly patient population.

Introduction

Periprosthetic fractures of the femur may occur during or after surgery. Intraoperative fractures are more likely to occur with press-fit and uncemented prostheses, and the reported incidence averages 1%. Postoperative periprosthetic fractures are associated with both cemented and uncemented stems (Fig. 1) and fall into two categories. They may happen when prosthetic loosening is present prior to the fracture and the femoral failure occurs within the area of osteolysis with a relatively minor trauma. At the other extreme, a substantial amount of force is necessary to fracture around a soundly fixed hip prosthesis. The quoted incidence for both scenarios averages 1%.

A variety of options are available to treat these fractures. Open reduction and internal fixation with compression plating and/or cerclage wiring is an attractive proposition when dealing with a fixed stem. Revision with morselised impacted bone grafting or even a structural allograft is being used if there is significant bone loss. Alternatively, revision with a long stem, especially using an uncemented press-fit technique, e. g. Wagner stem with tapered fins for anchoring in the distal femur, is an option when the bone stock is preserved.

In Belfast, we did not have the option of allograft, as our bone bank was established only recently. We therefore opted for the uncemented Kent hip system (Fig. 2) in cases of fractures around loose prostheses or intraoperative fractures during arthroplasty implantation. The use of this implant was also extended to some cases of neoplastic bone destruction. We see the Kent hip as a salvage procedure for those difficult situations when we need a combination of an intramedullary device and a hip prosthesis (Fig. 3).

We have analysed our early results and present our experience with this particular implant.

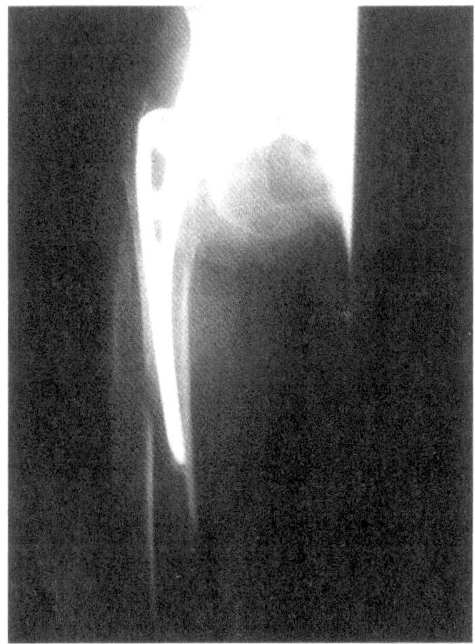

Fig. 1. Type II periprosthetic fracture around uncemented Austin-Moore hemiarthroplasty

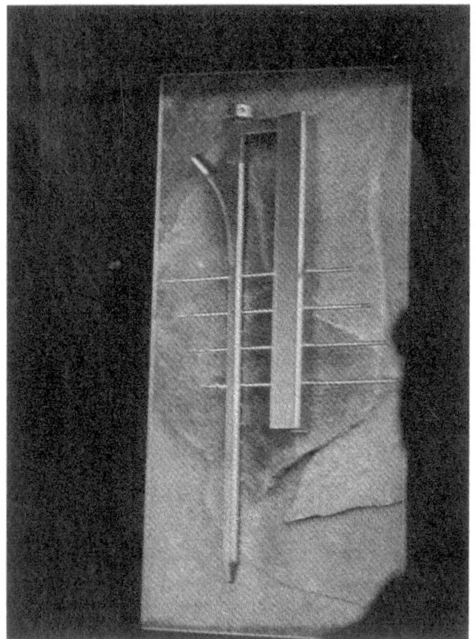

Fig. 2. Kent hip prosthesis with locking screws

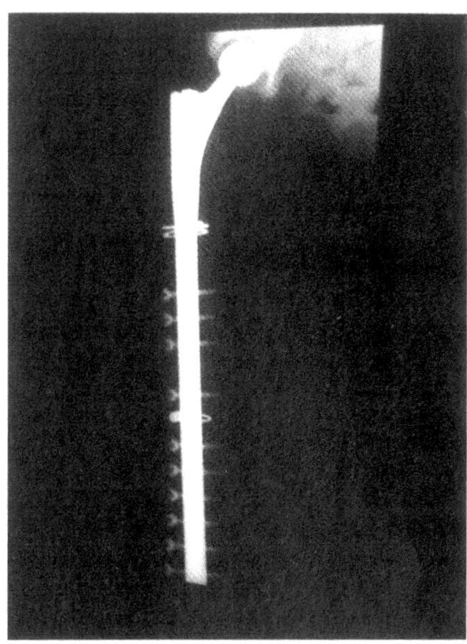

Fig. 3. Periprosthetic fracture fixed with Kent system and cerclage wires

Patients and Methods

From August 1993 to February 1996, 34 Kent hips were inserted into 33 consecutive patients in Belfast. Medical charts and radiographs were reviewed by one of the authors. Peroperative details, complications, and follow-up data were sought and analysed. Patients were reviewed on a yearly basis, wherever feasible.

Results

The distribution by sex was 21 women and 12 men. The mean age of the patients in our study was 78.5 years (range 55–91 years). The right femur was treated in 25 cases and the left in 9.

The indication for surgery was a periprosthetic fracture in 21 cases (Table 1). Of these, the primary prosthesis was a cemented total hip arthroplasty in all but 4 cases, where the periprosthetic fracture occurred around a hip hemiarthroplasty (Table 2).

Table 1. Indication for surgery

Acute periprosthetic fracture	21
Ununited fracture	5
Loose prosthetis	5
Pathological femur fracture	1
Loose + infected prothesis	1

Table 2. Distribution of primary protheses

Charnley total hip replacement	13
Howse total hip replacement	4
Monk hip hemiarthroplasty	2
Hastings hip hemiarthroplasty	1
Austin Moore hip hemiarthroplasty	1

Table 3. Types of periprosthetic fracture*

Type I	0
Zype II	9
Type III	12

* Johansson et al. classification.

Table 4. ASA* grading of patients

Grade 1	3
Grade 2	8
Grade 3	16
Grade 4	5
Grade 5	1

* American Society of Anaesthesiology.

The mean time from insertion of the primary prosthesis to fracture was 8.9 years (range 2 months to 20 years). The mean time from fracture to insertion of the Kent prosthesis was 9 days.

According to the classification by Johansson et al., where type I is a fracture at the stem of the prosthesis, type II a fracture at the tip of the prosthesis, and type III a fracture distal to the implant, our results showed a predominance of type III fractures (Table 3). Preoperatively, the majority of patients were classified as ASA grade 3 (Table 4).

The mean blood loss during the procedure amounted to 1990 ml (range 700–3620 ml). The total blood transfusion averaged 7.2 units (range 2–16 units). The mean operative time was 150 min (range 90–240 min).

All Kent hips were inserted via a posterior approach. Ten patients needed a Wagner-type osteotomy for cement removal, and all had at least 4 screws distal to the fracture. Fifteen of the 21 total hip arthroplasties needed replacement of the acetabular component, due to wear or loosening, while in the remaining 6 the acetabular cup was satisfactory and left in situ. One of the 4 hemiarthroplasties was converted to a total Kent arthroplasty.

The mean time of hospitalisation was on average 18.3 days. At discharge, 31 of the 33 patients were walking, although with aids. The place of discharge was to their own home for 19, other hospital for 9, care of elderly unit for 2 and a nursing home for 3 patients. In the immediate recovery period, one patient died on the 1st day due to myocardial infarction. Postoperative complications included 3 posterior dislocations, 1 prosthesis breached the anterior femoral cortex, 2 distal screw breakages, and in 1 patient the Kent

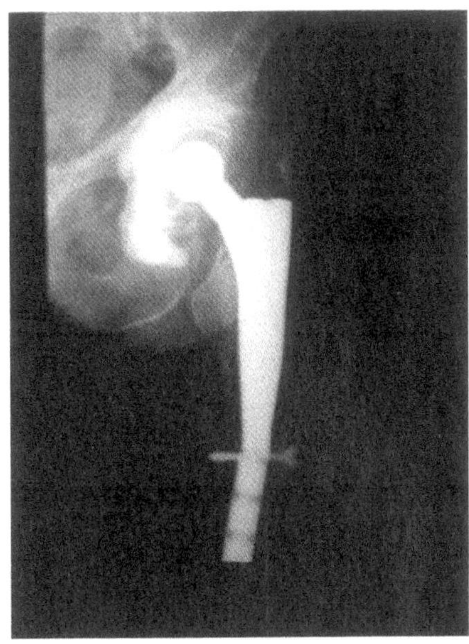

Fig. 4. Radiograph showing metal failure of
the Kent stem

stem failed and broke. Since then 9 patients have died and on annual follow-up of these patients, 2 further dislocations and a total of 1 non-union, 1 initial stem failure (Fig. 4) and 7 screw breakages occurred.

Discussion

Periprosthetic fractures can pose a significant challenge for a range of reasons. Technically, these fractures are difficult to fix with conventional open reduction and plating or cerclage wiring. Secondly, they often occur around an already loose stem, which will need revision, and on occasions the acetabular cup may need replacing, too. The type of population we deal with is elderly, often with significant medical problems and having difficulty ambulating. Therefore, the aim of any operation is to return these patients to their pre-fracture status. At the same time, the loosening of the prosthesis, which is causing discomfort around the hip, should be addressed.

We have found that the Kent hip works well under these circumstances and gives us the necessary flexibility to deal with the above-mentioned problems. The intramedullary device with locking screws permits early weight-bearing. This is crucial in these elderly patients to avoid postoperative complications due to recumbency. The hip replacement component of the Kent hip allows revision of the loose stem and accommodation of a previous socket.

We routinely use the posterior approach and often employ the Wagner-type osteotomy, which involves an osteotomy in the anteroposterior plane.

This greatly facilitates the removal of cement by allowing us to open the proximal femur like a book.

Straight long reamers are particularly helpful to prepare the curved medullary canal in order to accept the straight Kent stem. This reduces the incidence of anterior cortex perforation. After insertion of the Kent implant, the osteotomy is closed around its proximal stem with the help of cerclage wires or cables.

In most cases, the load is transferred to the distal locking screws, producing cortical thickening (Fig. 5), but we had 2 early screw failures, while the rest occurred within 18 months to 3 years of operation. In many cases these were inconsequential and were part of the subsidence, which accompanied closure of the fracture gap. We now recommend a minimum of 6 locking screws distal to the fracture, as well as proximal locking where possible, since our screw breakages were associated with a smaller number of distal screws.

Within this series there was one broken narrow size Kent stem at the level of the proximal locking screw hole. This has occurred in one other patient and is reported in a later series. The fact that the component is no longer manufactured of titanium, but of cobalt chrome, should reduce the incidence of stem failure in the future.

Once the Kent hip has provided initial temporary stability, its stem may require revision to a cemented stem of a more traditional configuration, after the fracture has healed (Fig. 6) and if a high demand is expected. This was the case in 2 of the patients in this series. One was a patient with lymphoma who suffered a pathological fracture of the femur, which responded to onco-

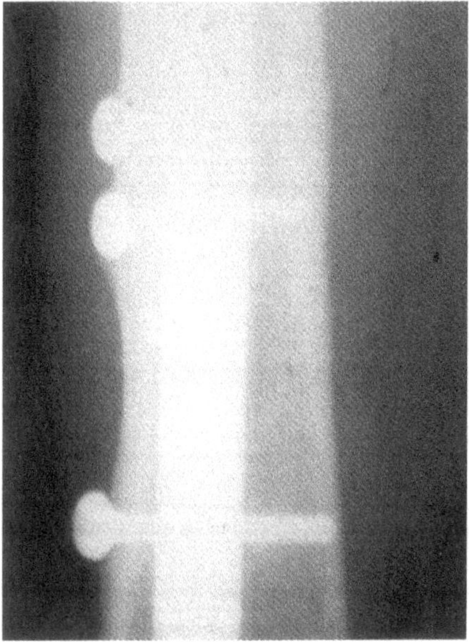

Fig. 5. Example of cortical hypertrophy due to load bearing

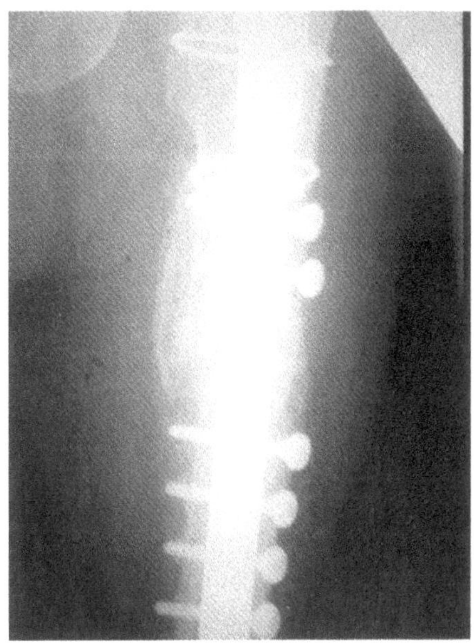

Fig. 6. Consolidated union across periprosthetic fracture treated with Kent hip

logical treatment, and the other was a farmer who continued to work despite insertion of a Kent hip.

We initially used 22-mm heads, which reflected our practice of inserting mainly Charnley total hip replacements as the primary procedure. We now use the 28-mm head, because it provides greater stability.

We have been very satisfied with the Kent hip and use it in about 50% of our periprosthetic fractures. Our main indication is a periprosthetic fracture in the elderly patient, for whom a period of traction would be deleterious. This patient requires early stabilisation, and due to the long-term low demand, they are able to mobilise early and regain relative independence. It is in our view a sound treatment for a fracture around the loose stem in which plating and/or cerclage wiring is contraindicated. Another problem for which the Kent hip offers a solution is a comminuted unstable fracture that requires length and rotational stability. With the increase in the number of total arthroplasties performed each year, the prevalence of periprosthetic fracture will probably increase and become a more frequently encountered problem.

Since this series, a prospective audit has been started to study the outcome in more detail and provide more information about long-term survivorship.

Reference

Johansson JE, McBroom R, Barrington TW, Hunter GA (1981) Fracture of the ipsilateral femur in patients with total hip replacement. J Bone Joint Surg 63 A:1435

V Antibiotic Loaded Bone Cements

Gentamicin Release from PMMA Bone Cement: Mechanism and Action on Bacteria

LARS FROMMELT

Introduction

Antibiotic-loaded bone cement (ALAC) is used widely today in the therapy of periprosthetic infection and other infectious conditions of bone tissue.

The success of ALAC is due to the special properties of polymethylmethacrylate (PMMA) polymer as a drug delivery system: appropriate substances can be eluted from the bone cement and are thus able to create concentrations which exceed those obtained by systemically administered antimicrobial agents.

The use of this principle goes back to the experiences of Buchholz and Lodenkämper in the early days of modern artificial joint replacement. At that time, the rate of periprosthetic infection following implantation of a joint prosthesis sometimes exceeded 10% [1, 2] and the systemic use of antimicrobial agents turned out to be ineffective against these infections without removal of the prosthesis. The concentrations at the site of infection were insufficient to act on the bacteria causing the infection.

From dental surgery, it was known that certain substances could be eluted from PMMA. Lodenkämper added several antimicrobial agents to PMMA bone cement in the laboratory and found that some of them were released over quite a long period of time. Especially gentamicin proved to be very effective in producing high concentrations for a long duration. Together with H. Engelbrecht [3], he carried out experiments in which the prophylactic use of gentamicin-loaded bone cement reduced the rate of infection to about 1% [4].

Later, Buchholz took the risk of using ALAC therapeutically for periprosthetic infection in a one-stage procedure with removal of the prosthesis and reimplantation of another artificial joint replacement.

Another approach to using ALAC for therapy was initiated by Klemm in Frankfurt [5]: he used beads of gentamicin-loaded bone cement threaded on a wire now known as Septopal® chain for the therapy of osteomyelitis.

Meanwhile, another application of ALAC was introduced: so-called spacers are formed with this material in two-stage revision arthroplasty for therapy of periprosthetic infection.

Antibiotic-loaded bone cement is used nowadays as a drug delivery system for both prophylaxis and therapy.

PMMA Bone Cement as a Drug Delivery System for Antimicrobial Agents

Initially the use of bone cement was – as in most cases in medicine – empirically based, with little knowledge of the underlying mechanisms.

Delivery of Antibiotics from PMMA Bone Cement In Vitro

One of the crucial properties of acrylic bone cement is that PMMA allows retention of antibiotics at the site of infection. This means that these substances can be applied in doses which would otherwise produce toxic side effects if not retarded by the delivery system. The key to understanding this mechanism is the knowledge of diffusion: the transport of substances follows the gradient from the highest to the lowest concentration in a system until the concentration is identical in all parts of that system. The time needed to balance the concentration depends on the mobility of the molecules involved. This works best if the substance is in a solvent, but diffusion is also possible in systems which are free of solvents. In such a system, the mobility of the molecules is rather slow and, in consequence, the substance is transported very slowly. Physicists call this a diffusion of masses.

Lindner [6], and later Low and coworkers [7], showed that the transport of antimicrobial agents in PMMA bone cement follows Fick's law and proved that it is really a kind of diffusion in the bone cement: this diffusion is free of solvents and takes place very slowly. This is how the antibiotics are transported to the bone cement surface, which is greatly enlarged by the porosity of the material.

When ALAC is incorporated in the human body, it is surrounded by an environment consisting mainly of water, which acts as a solvent. Thus, the velocity of diffusion increases tremendously, but at the same time the concentration diminishes with the third potential of the distance from the surface of the antibiotic-loaded PMMA. What looks like a great disadvantage at first glance turns out to be one of the outstanding features of this delivery system. High concentration is obtained at the site of infection while the concentration in the bloodstream remains 10^3 times lower than in the wound discharge at the beginning of therapy. Thus, side effects like nephrotoxicity can be avoided because the concentration at the site of adverse action, the renal tissue, remains very low.

The concentration of antibiotics produced by ALAC at the site of infection exceeds by many times the concentration that can be produced by any other route for administering antimicrobial agents. The concentration relates directly to the surface which is available for elution.

Several antimicrobial agents can be incorporated in PMMA bone cement, but not all agents are appropriate for this sort of application. They may not interact chemically with the bone cement. They have to remain stable at the temperatures generated by polymerisation of the PMMA. They must be able to perform mass diffusion in the PMMA matrix. At the moment, our knowledge about the conditions necessary for this behaviour is insufficient, so that we have to evaluate experimentally whether an antimicrobial agent is appropriate.

Delivery of Antibiotics from PMMA Bone Cement In Vivo

To evaluate clinical efficacy, it is necessary to look for the antibiotic concentration in the wound discharge at the site of implantation of the ALAC. In this context, a study by Adams and coworkers is of great relevance [8]. In an experiment performed on dogs, they showed that the concentrations of several antimicrobial agents exceed the minimal inhibitory concentrations (MIC) of several pathogens according to the National Committee for Clinical Laboratory Standards (NCCLS) breakpoints lasting from 3 to 38 days (Table 1).

Bacteria in Periprosthetic Infection

Specialised bacteria are able to colonise inorganic surfaces. If the surface belongs to a foreign body implanted in man, this may lead to a foreign body infection in the host.

The first step is the contamination of the foreign body and its colonisation. Concerning artificial joint replacement, this takes place at the interface between prosthesis and bone. The periprosthetic infection starts when the pathogen leaves the interface and induces osteomyelitis in the adjacent bone tissue. The onset of disease is delayed and it may be months or years before it becomes apparent, because the colonisation is characterised by the spread of bacteria along the surface of the foreign body at the interface [9,10].

Not only the host's condition is changed by the bacteria, the bacteria themselves change from planktonic to surface bond forms. This occurrence is characterised by the formation of glycocalix, a sort of slime which is the substrate of biofilm [11]. In this biofilm, the bacteria slow down their turnover and the duplication rate can be greatly extended (up to 20 h per cycle in staphylococci) [12]. Not only turnover may be altered, but also the genetic

Table 1. Detection of antimicrobial agents in wound discharge directly from PMMA bone cement (tibia of dogs) [8]

Antimicrobial agent	Period of release (days)	
	Concentration above breakpoint (NCCLS)	Concentration above 30 µg/ml
Cefazolin	14	>28
Ciprofloxacin	3	>28
Clindamycin	38	>28
Ticarcillin	9	>28
Tobramycin	21	>28
Vancomycin	3	>28

regulation: this may lead to a 100- to 800-fold increase in the minimal inhibitory concentration of antimicrobial agents in tobramycin compared with their planktonic forms, as shown by Costerton [13].

These data may explain why systemically administered antibiotics alone fail in the eradication of periprosthetic infection.

Clinical Use of Antibiotic-Loaded PMMA Bone Cement

Prophylaxis

Buchholz and coworkers demonstrated that ALAC is able to prevent periprosthetic infection [3].

To prevent artificial joint replacements from becoming infected, it is necessary to consider the pathogenesis of foreign body infection as previously described the first step towards periprosthetic infection is bacterial colonisation of the surface of the prosthetic system. In most cases this colonisation results from contamination during the surgical procedure for joint replacement [14].

If ALAC is used for fixation of the artificial joint, the surface is formed by the bone cement, which contains gentamicin. This antibiotic agent is able to prevent susceptible bacteria from colonising the foreign body. Thus, periprosthetic infection cannot develop.

It was demonstrated in vitro that the total time of delivery is longer than the period of detectable concentrations in the wound discharge. That means the antibiotics act for long time directly at the surface and are thus able to prevent colonisation. This effect of gentamicin may last for years, as demonstrated by Josefson [15] in a Swedish controlled prospective multicentre study. In this study, follow-up was at 1–2, 5, and 10 years. Up to 5 years after implantation, the number of infections was statistically significantly lower than in the group treated with systemic prophylaxis ($p>0.05$). There were 1,688 cases included in this study.

ALAC in Therapy

Encouraged by the success in prophylactic use, Buchholz and coworkers used antibiotic-loaded bone cement for the therapy of periprosthetic infection [2]. The essential factor for success in septic revision arthroplasty is the surgical procedure, with removal of all parts of the infected prosthetic system, including all bone cement, and radical debridement of all infected bone and soft tissue. After this surgical "cleaning", antibiotics are adjuvant but necessary for control of the infection, whether locally applied in bone cement or given intravenously.

Two-Stage Revision

In two-stage revision, the surgical procedure is performed as described above. After removal of the artificial joint replacement, a Girdlestone arthroplasty is performed and long-term systemic antibiotic therapy is carried out as in treatment of osteomyelitis. After the infection has been eliminated, a new prosthesis is implanted in a second surgical procedure [16].

A variant of this procedure is the use of ALAC as a so-called spacer. Because the concentration of antimicrobial agents in the bone following systemic application is low due to the pharmacokinetics of lower compartments, the use of drug delivery systems to obtain high concentrations at the site of infection was introduced. Antibiotic-loaded bone cement as a drug delivery system has the advantage that it can be used form devices that are able to fill the space left by removal of the prosthetic system, and thus the adverse effects on soft tissue by loss of distance (shrinking) can be avoided [17, 18].

Spacers must be removed because the delivery of drugs ceases after a certain period of time depending on the antibiotics used. What remains after the antibiotics are gone is a foreign body at risk of colonisation by bacteria but without the positive effects for the patient that result from artificial joint replacement.

One-Stage Revision

In one-stage revision, the infected prosthesis is removed in the same manner, but after surgical "cleaning" another prosthesis is implanted during the same operation. This is possible because of the use of ALAC, which forms the surface of the prosthetic system and is thus able to prevent remaining bacteria in the situs from recolonising the artificial joint replacement. The function of ALAC is not only to produce a high concentration of antibiotics locally but to form a barrier against bacterial colonisation of the surface [19].

The crucial factor in one-stage revision is that the pathogen must be known before surgery so that the antibiotics added to the bone cement can be chosen according to individual susceptibility testing. The selection of the antimicrobial agents depends not only on the susceptibility of the pathogen but also on their properties of elution from the PMMA bone cement and whether these agents are available in appropriate form (Table 2).

Some rules have to be respected if antibiotics are added to bone cement in the operating theatre. Antibiotics can be used only as a powder, and this has to be mixed carefully with the polymer powder of the PMMA. The mixture

Table 2. Examples of dosage of antimicrobial agents for local application in PMMA bone cement. Maximum dosage for clinical use: 4 g antimicrobial agents per 40 g PMMA (stability of bone cement!)

1.0 g Clindamycin	1.0 g gentamicin	
2.0 g Vancomycin	1.0 g ampicillin	1.0 g gentamicin
2.0 g Cefazedon	1.0 g gentamicin	
2.0 g Cefotaxim	1.0 g gentamicin	
2.0 g Vancomycin	1.0 g ofloxacin	1.0 g gentamicin
2.0 g Cefoperazon	2.0 g amikacin	

should be as homogeneous as possible. Whenever available, industrial preparations should be used because they are superior to any hand-made preparation with respect to elution properties and stability of the bone cement. Unfortunately, many antibiotics necessary for the control of periprosthetic infection are not available in such preparations. This applies to one-stage revision and the use of spacers as well.

Conclusions

Antimicrobial agents added to PMMA bone cement are effective in infections of bone tissue with or without foreign bodies and of little harm to the patient if used as indicated in addition to radical and meticulous surgery.

If ALAC is used as a drug delivery system, the antibiotics used must be effective against the pathogens involved. This system is able to realise high concentrations at the site of infection, whether used for fixation of a prosthesis, as a spacer, or in beads as introduced by Klemm. If used for prosthesis fixation, ALAC is effective as a barrier against recolonisation of the surface of the system.

The efficacy of ALAC depends on the homogeneity of the mixture of PMMA and antibiotics; therefore industrial mixes are superior to hand-made preparations.

References

1. Charnley J (1964) A clean-air operating enclosure. Brit J Surgery 51:195–202
2. Buchholz HW, Elson RA, Engelbrecht E, Lodenkämper H, Röttger J, Siegel A (1981) Management of deep infection of total hip replacement. J Bone Joint Surg 63B:342–353
3. Buchholz HW, Engelbrecht H (1970) Über die Depotwirkung einiger Antibiotika bei Vermischung mit dem Kunstharz Palacos. Chirurg 41:511–515
4. Buchholz HW, Elson RA, Lodenkämper H (1979) The infected joint implant. In: McKibbin B (ed) Recent Advances in Orthopaedics 3. Churchill Livingston, New York, pp. 139–161
5. Klemm K (1979) Gentamicin-PMMA-Kugeln in der Behandlung abszedierender Knochen- und Weichteilinfektionen. Zbl Chir 104:934–942
6. Lindner B (1981) Physikalische Analyse des Freisetzungsmechanismus von Chemotherapeutika aus dotiertem Polymethylmetacrylat. Inauguraldissertation. Kiel, Germany
7. Low HT, Fleming RH, Gilmore MFX, McCarthy ID, Hughes SPF (1986) In vitro measurement and computer modelling of the diffusion of antibiotic in bone cement. J Biomed Eng 8:149–155
8. Adam K, Couch L, Cierny G, Calhoun J, Mader JT (1992) In vitro and in vivo evaluation of antibiotic-impregnated polymethylmethacrylate beads. Clin Orthop 278:244–252
9. Gristina AG (1987) Biomaterial-centered infection: microbial adhesion versus tissue integration. Science 237:1588–1595
10. Frommelt L (2000) Periprosthetic infection – bacteria and the interface between prosthesis and bone. In: Learmonth ID (ed) Interfaces in total hip arthroplasty. Springer, London
11. Brisou JF (1995) Biofilms – methods of enzymatic release of micro organisms. CRC Press, Boca Raton
12. Zak O, Sande MA (1982) Correlation of in vitro activity of antibiotics with results of treatment in experimental animal models and human infection. In: Sabath LD (ed) Action of antibiotics in patients. Hans Huber Publishers, Bern, pp. 55–67

13. Costerton JW, Lewandowski Z, Caldwell DE, Korber DR, Lappin-Scott HM (1995) Microbial biofilms. Annu Rev Microbiol 49:711–745
14. Lidwell OM (1988) Air, antibiotics and sepsis in replacement joints. J Hosp Inf 11 [Suppl C]:18–40
15. Josefson G, Kolmert L (1993) Prophylaxis with systemic antibiotics versus gentamicin bone cement in total hip arthroplasty. A ten-year survey of 1,688 hips. Clin Orthop 292:210–214
16. McDonald DJ, Fitzgerald RH, Ilstrup DM (1989) Two-stage reconstruction of a total hip arthroplasty because of infection. J Bone Joint Surg 71-A:828–834
17. McMaster WC (1995) Technique for intraoperative construction PMMA spacers in total knee revision. Am J Orthop 24:178–180
18. Oxborrow NJ, Stamer J, Andrews M, Stone MH (1997) New uses for gentamicin impregnated polymethyl methacrylate in two-stage revision hip arthroplasty. J Arthroplasty 12:709–710
19. Steinbrink K, Frommelt L (1995) Behandlung der periprothetischen Infektion der Hüfte durch einzeitige Austauschoperation. Orthopäde 24:335–343

Pharmacokinetic Study of a Gentamicin/Clindamicin Bone Cement Used in One-stage Revision Arthroplasty

THORSTEN GEHRKE, GÖTZ VON FÖRSTER, LARS FROMMELT

Abstract. Gram-positive organisms, primarily *Staphylococcus aureus* and *epidermidis*, continue to be the organisms most frequently responsible for infected joint prostheses. We investigated a new bone cement containing 1 g gentamicin and 1 g clindamycin per 40 g Palacos. The purpose of this prospective in vivo study was to measure the elution of gentamicin and clindamycin antibiotics from Palacos bone cement in one-stage hip revision arthroplasty. The study was performed on 24 patients who were suffering from infected total hip replacements. Venous blood samples, drainage fluid and urine were collected from each patient before and up to 10 days after operation. The average concentration in the drainage fluid was more than 100 times higher than in the serum. All infections were treated successfully. No recurrence or persistence of the periprosthetic infection was reported and no side-effects were observed during the first postoperative year.

Introduction

Periprosthetic infection is a severe complication following artificial joint replacement. It is a failure for the surgeon and a catastrophe for the patient. Periprosthetic infection must be clearly differentiated from other bone infections such as osteomyelitis because a foreign body is involved. This kind of infection follows the rules of a foreign body infection. If a foreign body is involved there is a typical interaction between the foreign body and the bacteria that are able to colonize it as described by Gristina and co-workers (1985): in the very early stages of colonization, immediately after contamination of the prosthetic device, bacterial growth begins with the formation of slime, the "biofilm", followed by a dramatic prolongation of the generation time. Signs of infection may occur very late, when the bacteria leave the interface, invade surrounding tissue and induce a secondary osteomyelitis.

Under these conditions therapy with systemic antibiotics will fail if the prosthesis is not removed. There are two main approaches in the surgical treatment of periprosthetic infection: one-stage or two-stage exchange revision.

In the ENDO-Klinik in Hamburg more than 6000 septic revisions have been performed during the last 25 years by using the one-stage revision procedure. The two most important features of this procedure are removal of the infected prosthesis and radical debridement of all infected tissue.

Reimplantion of a new artificial joint in the same operation is possible when antibiotic loaded acrylic bone cement is used for fixation, because extremely high concentrations of antibiotics at the surface of the newly implanted device are able to prevent its colonization by bacteria. The use of antibiotic-impregnated cement for fixation of prosthetic implants in bone was first reported by Buchholz and Engelbrecht in 1970. A number of studies have shown the biomechanical effect and antimicrobial activity of several antibiotics in bone cement, particularly gentamicin.

This kind of cement allows retention of the antibiotics at the site of infection. The transport of antimicrobial agents within the bone cement is free of solvent and therefore it takes place very slowly. Once the antibiotics reach the surface of the bone cement their concentration diminishes with the third potency of the distance by diffusion in the bloodstream.

However, there are some rules that have to be respected when antibiotics are added to bone cement in the operation room. Antibiotics can be used only in powder form and the mixture must be as homogenous as possible. The antibiotic must be stable in the presence of high temperatures and the concentration of the antibiotics in the bone cement should not be more than 10% of the whole mass of bone cement. For example, the volume of antibiotic powder in 40 g cement should not be more than 4 g.

Our earlier studies have shown that this method, employing only a single operation, is successful in more than 87% of cases. Up to now we have always added a specific antibiotic, depending on the susceptibility of the bacteria, to the Refobacin Palacos bone cement by hand. With this procedure, however, a homogeneous mixture and the required sterile conditions are not always achievable. We have therefore developed a new bone cement in co-operation with the Merck company. This industrially manufactured bone cement contains 1 g clindamycin and 1 g gentamicin per 40 g cement. Gentamicin is an aminoglycoside with a bactericidal effect. Clindamycin belongs to the lincosamine group and has a predominantly bacteriostatic effect on gram-positive bacteria such as staphylococci and streptococci, Gram-positive anaerobes such as peptostreptococci, and also on Gram-negative anaerobes (e.g. bacteroides).

Materials and Methods

In a prospective controlled study we investigated the pharmacokinetic properties of the antibiotics gentamicin and clindamycin in bone cement and the clinical outcome after 12 months. Twenty-four patients (8 female, 16 male) were eligible for the study. The average age was 59 years (20–78 years). All had had periprosthetic infection at the hip, which had been diagnosed by means of preoperative joint aspiration. In most cases the causative organisms were staphylococci or streptococci.

All patients underwent one-stage exchange arthroplasty. The new implant was fixed in position using industrially manufactured antibiotic-loaded bone cement containing 1 g gentamicin and 1 g clindamycin per 40 g polymethyl-methacrylate (PMMA).

Samples of venous blood, wound fluid and urine were collected for up to 10 days after the operation. The antibiotic concentrations were measured by the inhibition activity in the Agar-Diffusion-Test described by Grove and Randel (1955) by using test organisms, each of which were susceptible to only one of the two antibiotics. The detection limit of both antibiotics was 0.04 µg/ml.

The outcome and effectiveness of the therapy were evaluated by serial radiographs, laboratory data and clinical examination 6 and 12 months post-operatively. This included determination of the patient's hip score according to Merle d'Aubigné.

Results

Serum Concentrations of Gentamicin and Clindamycin (Fig. 1)

Thirty minutes after implantation of the new hip prosthesis the mean genta-micin concentration in the serum was 0.96 µg/ml. After 2 h it was 0.87 µg/ml, and after 6 h 0.47 µg/ml. One day after implantation the level was only 0.13 µg/ml and on the second day 0.001 µg/ml. On the third day it was no longer possible to detect gentamicin in the serum.

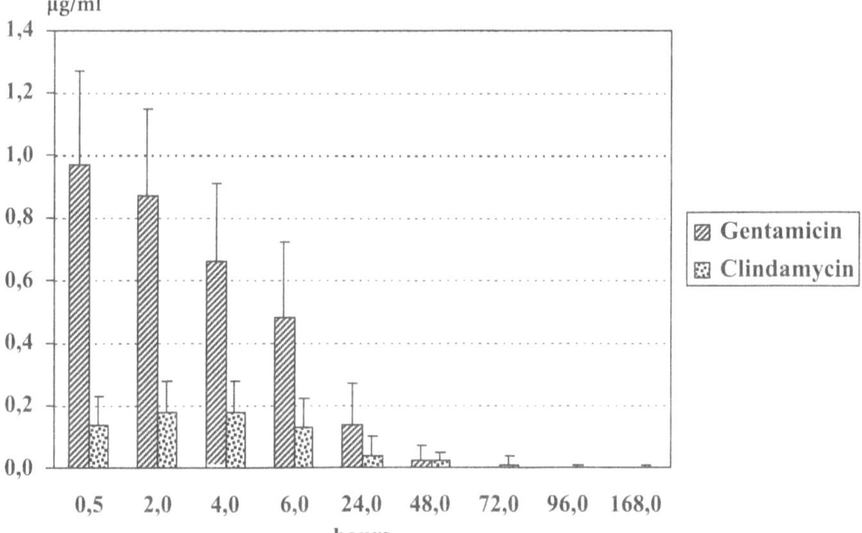

Fig. 1. Serum concentration

The mean clindamycin concentration in the serum was 0.14 µg/ml at 30 min after implantation, 0.18 µg/ml after 2 h, and 0.13 µg/ml after 6 h. One day after implantation it was only 0.04 µg/ml and on the second and third days 0.01 µg/ml. From the fourth postoperative day clindamycin could no longer be detected in the serum.

Gentamicin and Clindamycin Concentrations in Wound Fluid

In the wound fluid yielded by the drains from the wound cavity the mean gentamicin concentration was 28.74 µg/ml on the first postoperative day and 18.61 µg/ml on the second. The mean clindamycin concentration from the wound fluid was 28.97 µg/ml on the first postoperative day and 26.03 µg/ml on the second (Fig. 2).

Gentamicin and Clindamycin Concentrations in Urine

The mean value of gentamicin elimination fell quickly from 10.91 µg/ml on the first postoperative day to 2.71 µg/ml on the second day and further to 1.17 µg/ml on the tenth postoperative day. The results for the elimination of clindamycin were similar. On the first day the concentration was 2.35 µg/ml, on the second 0.86 µg/ml and finally on the tenth day 0.15 µg/ml (Fig. 3).

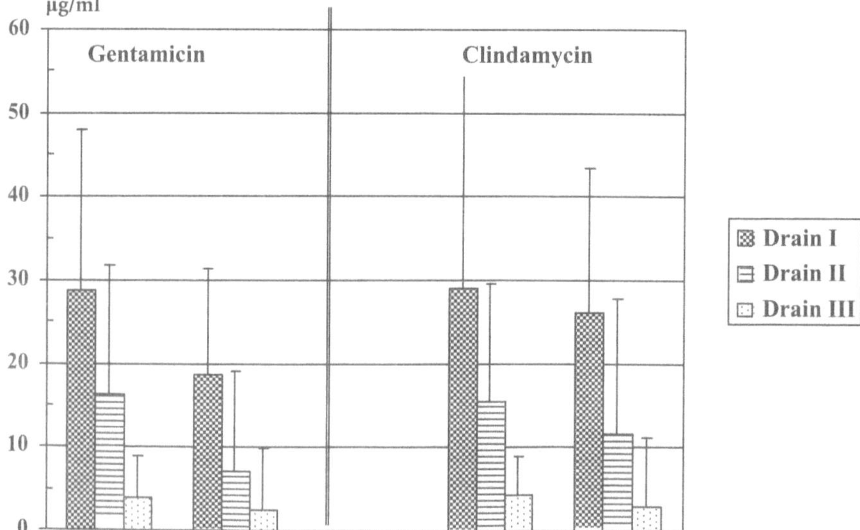

Fig. 2. Concentration in wound drainage fluid

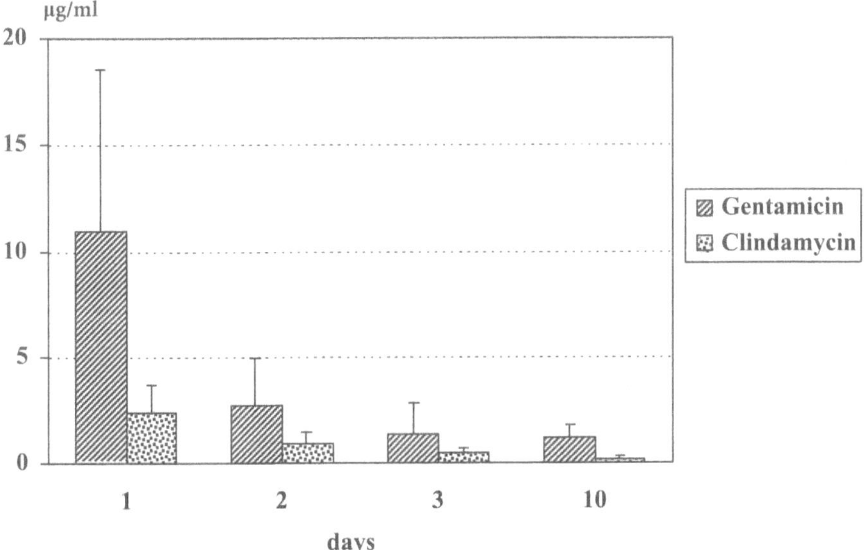

Fig. 3. Urine concentration

Recovery Rate

The recovery rate in the serum and urine was evidence of a continuous elution from the bone cement similar to that observed in previous laboratory experiments (Fig. 3). The results obtained from wound fluid in the first two postoperative days showing an average of 0.92% for gentamicin and 0.99% for clindamycin are comparable.

The average recovery rate in urine (Fig. 4) during the first 10 postoperative days was 2.221 for gentamicin and 0.54 for clindamycin. This clear difference is due to the different metabolization of the two substances.

Clinical Results

After the first postoperative year none of the patients showed signs of recurrence or persistence of infection, nor were there any antibiotic-related side-effects. Clinical results based on Merle d'Aubigné's hip score showed a significant improvement with regard to pain (preoperative: 2.2, postoperative: 5.2), walking ability (preoperative: 2.2, postoperative: 5.0), and function (preoperative: 2.5, postoperative: 5.4) (Fig. 5). Analysis of the radiographs after 1 year showed that none of the patients had any signs of loosening. Laboratory testing of infection parameters did not reveal a rise in values for any of the patients.

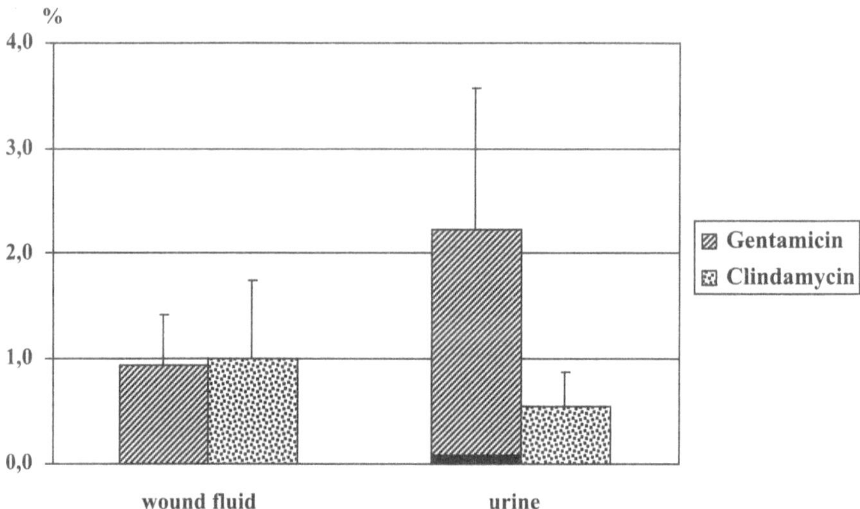

Fig. 4. Recovery rate

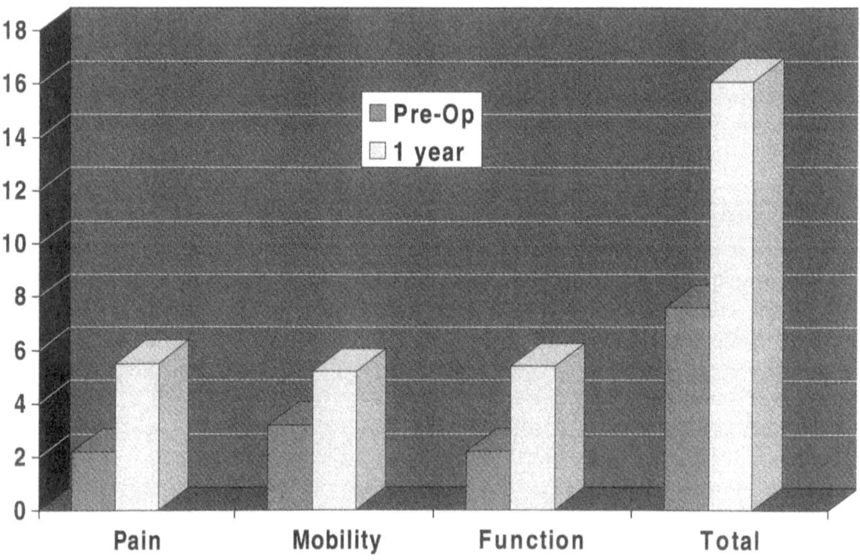

Fig. 5. Clinical Results (Merle d'Aubigne)

Discussion

The use of antibiotic-loaded bone cement can only be successful when the antibiotic concentration in the serum is below the toxicity level but at the same time high enough to have a bactericidal effect in the environment of the implant and thus prevent re-colonization of the implant surface. Thirty minutes after implantation the gentamicin concentration in the serum was 0.96 µg/ml, it then fell to 0.13 µg/ml on the first postoperative day and fell further to 0.01 µg/ml on the second day. By the third postoperative day gentamicin could no longer be detected in the serum. Experiments have shown that damage to the renal tubules only occurs if the serum concentrations lie above 0.2 µg/ml for a longer period. A nephrotoxic effect following the use of gentamicin-impregnated bone cement is therefore not to be expected. This was confirmed by the absence of side-effects in the patients in the study.

The elution of clindamycin corresponded largely to that of gentamicin with regard to both concentration and duration. These two antibiotics therefore show similar elution properties when mixed with bone cement in the same concentration.

This corresponds to in vitro studies by Cimbollek (1994) during which the same amounts of gentamicin sulphate and clindamycin hydrochloride were added to the cement. The results showed that both antibiotics were eluted in equal quantities and with equal speed.

Both pharmacokinetic and clinical results of the 1-year follow-up study are evidence of the effectiveness of adding a combination of gentamicin and clindamycin to bone cement. Tests revealed that there was a high local concentration of the antibiotics with continuous elution from the bone cement while systemic levels remained low. Side-effects were not observed. There was no persistence or recurrence of the periprosthetic infection after 1 year. The medium-term clinical results show that sufficient mechanical stability was achieved, comparable to that of Refobacin-Palacos®, and that antibiotic-loaded bone cement is a useful addition in surgical procedures because it can prevent re-colonization of newly implanted devices. The type of surgical procedure chosen to treat periprosthetic infection, whether one-stage or two-stage, is not important. The factors that are decisive for the success of the procedure are the proven susceptibility of the pathogens to clindamycin and gentamicin plus radical debridement. The combination of clindamycin and gentamicin is the most appropriate antibiotic weapon in such cases because most pathogens causing periprosthetic infections have a susceptibility pattern covered by these agents.

References

1. Begg EJ, Peddi BA, Chambers ST, Boswell DR (1992) Comparison of gentamicin dosing regimens using an in-vitro model. J Antimicrob Chemother 29:427–433
2. Buchholz HW, Engelbrecht H (1970) Über die Depotwirkung einiger Antibiotika bei Vermischung mit dem Kunstharz Palacos. Chirurg 41:511–515
3. Buchholz HW, Elson RA, Engelbrecht E, Lodenkämper H, Röttger J, Siegel A (1981) Management of deep infection of total hip replacement. J Bone Joint Surg 63-B:342–353
4. Cimbollek M (1994) Entwicklung einer antibiotikageschützten Herzklappe zur Prophylaxe und Therapie der künstlichen Endokarditis. Pharmazeutische Dissertation. J.W. Goethe-Universität, Frankfurt a.M
5. Dingeldein E (1989) Mikrobiologische Untersuchungen mit Gentamicin und Clindamycin. E. Merck, Darmstadt, EMD 55:201
6. Espehaug B, Engesaeter LB, Vollset SE, Havelin LI, Langeland N (1997) Antibiotic prophylaxis in total hip arthroplasty. Review of 10,905 primary cemented total hip replacements reported to the Norwegian arthroplasty register, 1987 to 1995. J Bone Joint Surg [Br] 79-4:590–595
7. Frommelt L, Heinert K, Lodenkämper H, Buchholz HW (1988) Lincomycin/gentamicin-loaded PMMA-bone-cement in the management of deep infection of total hip replacement by one stage exchange arthroplasty. Proceedings of the 4th International Congress on Clinical Microbiology, Nice, Abstract S40
8. Gehrke T, v. Foerster G, Frommelt L, Marx A (1996) Elution properties of a gentamicin-clindamycin impregnated bone cement in one stage revision arthroplasty. Orthop Trans 20:68
9. Gristina A (1987) Biomaterial centered infection: microbial adhesion versus tissue integration. Science 237:1588–1595
10. Gristina A, Costerton JW (1984) Bacterial adherence, the glycocalix and musculoskeletal sepsis. Orthop Clin North Am 15:517–535
11. Grove DC, Randall AW (1955) Assay methods of antibiotics. Medical Encyclopedia Inc., New York
12. Joseffsson G, Gudmundsson G, Kolmert L, Wijkström S (1990) Prophylaxis with systemic antibiotics versus gentamicin bone cement in total hip arthroplasty. Clin Orthop Rel Res 253:173–178
13. Klüber D (1985) Konzentrationsmessungen von Clindamycin und Clindamycin-Gentamicin-Kombinationen nach Beimengung zum Knochenzement Palacos R. Med Inauguaral-dissertation, Universität Hamburg
14. Landuyt VHW (1987) Spectrum of clindamycin: in vitro effects and efficiacy. Acta Therapeutica 13:541–552
15. Lodenkämper H, Lodenkämper U, Trompa K (1982) Über die Ausscheidung von Antibiotika aus dem Knochenzement Palacos. Z Ortop 120:801–805
16. Masri BA, Duncan CP, Beauchamp CP (1996) Long term elution of antibiotics from bone cement: an in vivo study using the Prostalac system. Orthop Trans 20:69
17. Salvati EA, Callaghan JJ, Brause BD, Rimnac CM, Wright TM (1987) Reimplantation in infection: elution of gentamicin from cement and beads. Clin Orthop 207:83–96
18. Steinbrink K, Frommelt L (1995) Behandlung der periprothetischen Infektion der Hüfte durch einzeitige Austauschoperation. Orthopäde 24:335–343
19. Wahlig H, Dingeldein E, Bergmann R, Reuss K (1978) The release of gentamicin from PMMA beads. An experimental and pharmacokinetic study. J Bone Joint Surg 60-B:270
20. Wahlig H, Dingeldein E, Buchholz HW, Buchholz M, Bachmann F (1984) Pharmakokinetic study of gentamicin-loaded cement in total hip replacements. Comparative effects of varying dosage. J Bone Joint Surg 66-B:174–179
21. Wilson DH (1980) Clindamycin in the treatment of soft tissue infections: a review of 15 019 patients. Br J Surg 67:93

Effect of Type of Bone Cement and Antibiotic Prophylaxis on Early Revision of Cemented Total Hip Replacement Presentation from the Norwegian Arthroplasty Register 1987–1996

OVE FURNES, LEIF IVAR HAVELIN, BIRGITTE ESPEHAUG

Introduction

The Norwegian Orthopaedic Association took the initiative to establish the Norwegian Hip Register in 1987. The background to this was the well-known disaster of the Christiansen (Sudmann et al. 1983) and resurfacing prostheses (Howie et al. 1990). Due to the poor results of these prostheses, many Norwegian orthopaedic surgeons started using undocumented, uncemented prostheses. The register's main purpose was to help detect inferior implants as early as possible. After about 3 years, we observed inferior results with uncemented implants compared to cemented ones. This difference was the largest in young patients (Havelin et al. 1994). The overall short-term results of the most commonly used cemented total hip prostheses were found to be good, with a 5-year revision probability of 2.5% (Espehaug et al. 1995). However, in short-term results, the type of cement seems to be more important than the type of prosthesis. This paper presents published results on the effect on early prosthesis survival of type of bone cement and antibiotic prophylaxis.

Materials and Methods

After each primary hip replacement operation, Norwegian orthopaedic surgeons fill in a one-page form with information concerning operating technique, including accurate descriptions of all implant parts and cement types (Havelin et al. 1993). If the prosthesis is revised later, possibly at another hospital, we receive a new report with information about the reason for and type of revision. Using the patient's national social security number, revisions are linked to the primary operations. We receive information from the Norwegian Population Registry on dates of patient deaths. Differences in patient material are handled by adjusting with multiple regression analyses (Cox 1972) or by limiting materials to homogeneous subgroups and using Kaplan-Meier survival analysis (Kaplan, Meier 1958). The studies presented have follow-ups from September 1987 until January 1994 or January 1996. The endpoint (failure) in the survival analyses is revision surgery.

Results

Study 1 (Havelin et al. 1995)

The aim of this study was to compare the results of total hip arthroplasty with respect to different cement types and viscosity and the addition of an antibiotic to the cement. A total of 8579 primary Charnley total hip replacements were studied from 1987 to 1993. The reason for operation was primary coxarthrosis, and no previous operation in the index hip was allowed. The endpoint was aseptic loosening of one or both of the acetabular and femoral components. All types of cement used in Norway were investigated. The number of cemented hips with the different cement types are given in Table 1. Figure 1 shows significantly better results with high-viscosity cements after 5 years than with low-viscosity cements (CMW 3), and after only 2 years the Boneloc cement had significantly worse results than high-viscosity cements. The risk ratios are given in Table 2. At 5 years, there was no significant difference between the three high-viscosity cements.

Study 2 (Espehaug et al. 1997)

This study compares the effect on implant survival of the different regimes of antibiotic prophylaxis used for hip arthroplasty in Norway, particularly with regard to the possible benefit of adding antibiotics to bone cement. The

Table 1. Cemented Charnley prostheses for primary coxarthrosis reported to the Norwegian Arthroplasty Register 1987–1993 [7]

Cement type	Viscosity	Manufacturer	n
Palacos	High	Schering-Plough	1037
Palacos with gentamicin	High	Schering-Plough	2775
CMW 1	High	DePuy	2309
CMW 3	Low	DePuy	1193
Simplex	High	Howmedica	435
Boneloc	Cold curing	Polymers Reconstructive	764
Others			66

Table 2. Cemented Charnley prostheses reported to the Norwegian Arthroplasty Register 1987–1993 showing relative risk of revision due to aseptic loosening as determined by the Cox regression model and adjusted for gender and age [7]

Viscosity/cement	Cox risk ratio (95% CI)
High, without antibiotic	1
High, with antibiotic	0.6 (0.4–1.0)
Low	2.5 (1.6–3.9)
Boneloc	8.5 (4.9–14.5)

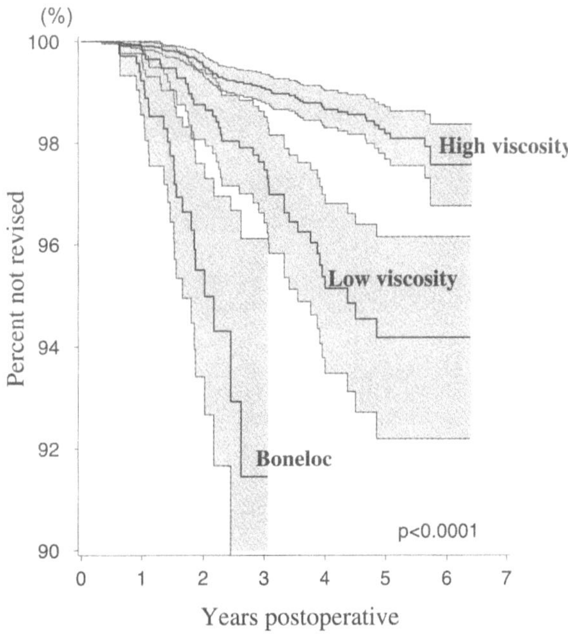

Fig. 1. Kaplan-Meier survival curves of Charnley femoral prostheses with high-viscosity, low-viscosity, and Boneloc cements. From the Norwegian Arthroplasty Register 1987–1993, a study of 8579 primary cemented Charnley femoral prosthesis in primary coxarthrosis (reproduced with permission [7])

study was based on 10 905 primary cemented total hip replacements operated on for coxarthrosis and with no previous operation in the index hip. The material included four different prosthesis brands: Charnley (DePuy, Leeds, UK) (55%), Exeter (Howmedica International, Herouville, France) (20%), Titan (Landos, Chaumont, France) (16%), and Spectron/ITH (cup/stem) (Richards, Memphis, Tenn., USA) (10%). The high-viscosity cements included were Palacos without antibiotic (Schering-Plough International, Kenilworth, N.J., USA) (18%), Simplex without antibiotic (Howmedica International, London, UK) (27%), Palacos with gentamicin (Schering-Plough) (54%), and Simplex with erythromycin/colistin (1%). Four different prophylaxis regimens were investigated: (1) with systemic antibiotic and antibiotic in the cement (5804 hips), (2) with systemic antibiotic prophylaxis only (4586 hips), (3) with antibiotic-containing cement only (239 hips), and (4) with no antibiotic prophylaxis (276 hips). Figure 2 shows the survival curves for prostheses with the four regimens with any revision as endpoint. In Table 3, risk ratios are given for the four treatment groups, with revision caused by deep infection as endpoint. The figure and the table both show significantly better survival in the group with both systemic antibiotic and antibiotic-containing cement.

Table 3. Cemented Charnley prosthesis reported to the Norwegian Arthroplasty Register 1987–1995 showing relative risk of revision due to deep infection as estimated by the Cox regression model, with adjustment for gender, age, cement, prosthesis brand, type of operating theatre, and operating time [3]

Treatment regimen	Cox risk ratio (95 CI)
Systemic antibiotic and antibiotic in cement	1
Systemic only	4.3 (1.7–11), $p=0.001$
Antibiotic in cement only	6.3 (1.6–25), $p=0.003$
No antibiotic	11.5 (2.1–63), $p=0.002$

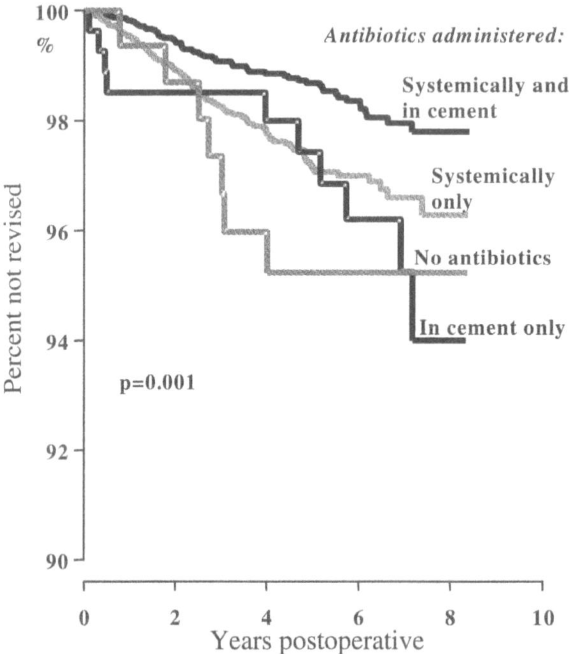

Fig. 2. Cox regression adjusted survival curves of total hip replacements performed in Norway 1987–1995. The probabilities of survival were calculated for patients receiving different antibiotic regimens for prophylaxis, with revision due to any cause as endpoint. The p value refers to a homogeneity test showing a statistically significant difference in survival between the regimens (reproduced with permission [3])

Study 3 (Furnes et al. 1997)

This study examined the 5-year results of Boneloc cement with Charnley prostheses and investigated whether the inferior results also applied to the Exeter prosthesis. Under study were 172 Exeter and 955 Charnley prostheses fixated with Boneloc cement and 6621 Charnley and 1645 Exeter prostheses cemented with high-viscosity cement (CMW 1, Palacos, and Simplex). Follow-up was at 0–5 years. Both Charnley and Exeter prostheses had significantly better survival results with high-viscosity cemented components than with Boneloc-cemented components. Boneloc-cemented Charnley femoral components showed a 14-fold higher risk of revision than high-viscosity cemented components (Fig. 3), and an Exeter femoral component had seven times more risk of revision than with the use of high-viscosity cement. Exeter prostheses cemented with Boneloc had better results than Charnley prostheses using Boneloc (Fig. 4).

Discussion

Study 1

We showed that, after only 2 years' follow-up of Charnley prostheses, Boneloc cement had inferior results compared to high-viscosity cement brands and, after 5 years, the CMW 3 low-viscosity cement showed inferior results. Boneloc cement was introduced to the Norwegian and international markets with only laboratory tests as documentation. There had been no clinical or randomised studies to support the laboratory results. In laboratory tests and clini-

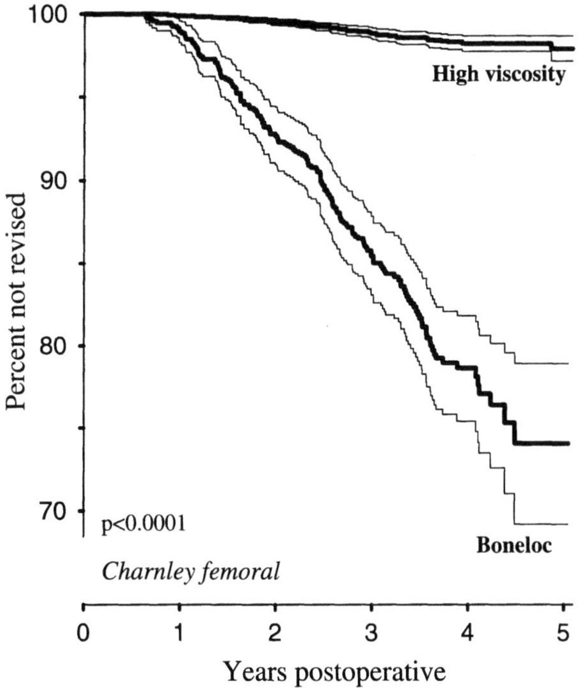

Fig. 3. Kaplan-Meier analyses of revision due to aseptic loosening. Boneloc-cemented and high-viscosity-cemented Charnley femoral components are compared. The *p* value refers to a log rank test of differences between the curves in survival. From the Norwegian Arthroplasty Register 1991–1995 (reproduced with permission [4])

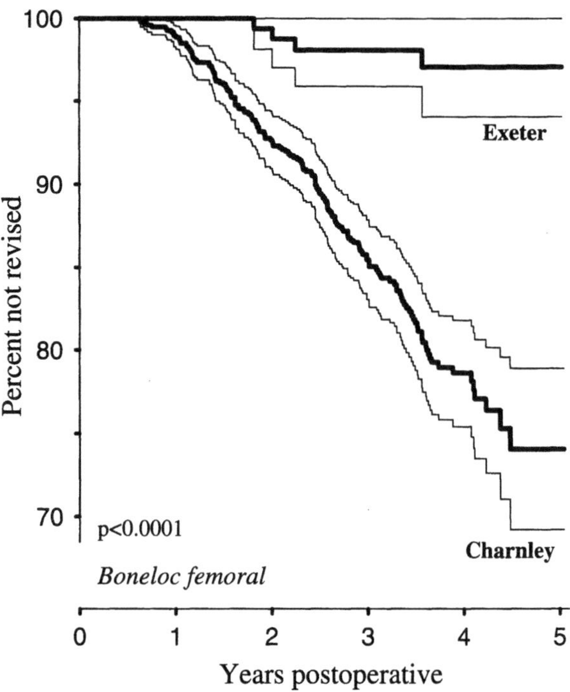

Fig. 4. Kaplan-Meier analyses of revision due to aseptic loosening. Boneloc-cemented Charnley and Exeter femoral components are compared. The *p* value refers to a log rank test of differences between the curves in survival. From the Norwegian Arthroplasty Register 1991–1995 (reproduced with permission [4])

cal roentgen stereophotogrammetric analysis (RSA), Tanner et al. (1995) showed that the Boneloc cement provided fixation of both the acetabulum and femoral components inferior to that with standard high-viscosity cement. Experience with Boneloc shows that the results of new cements should be documented through both laboratory tests and randomised clinical studies with the RSA technique (Nilsson, Kärholm 1996) before being introduced to the market (Malchau 1995). The use of CMW 3 low-viscosity cement is extensive internationally, although its has been stopped in Norway. It has been argued that the results of low-viscosity cement in laboratory tests are good and that the inferior clinical results with CMW 3 are due to bad cementing technique. Many orthopaedic surgeons find, however, that low-viscosity cement is difficult to use, and arguments for its use should be based on good, documented clinical results.

Study 2

The second study showed that antibiotic prophylaxis administered both systemically and in the cement resulted in fewer revisions than the other regimens, with endpoint being revision due to any cause. The reason for the previous finding could be that some aseptic loosenings are in fact low-grade septic loosenings and that the combined antibiotic regimen also prevented some of these loosenings. Randomised trials have compared the effect of antibiotics in the bone cement to those with antibiotics given systemically (Josefsson et al. 1981, 1990, 1993; McQueen et al. 1990), but the results were inconclusive, with no difference reported in the smallest study (McQueen 1990) and no statistically significant improvement in the rate of deep infection in the hips with antibiotic-containing cement (Josefsson 1993).

Study 3

This study had a longer follow-up on Boneloc cement and confirmed the previously reported inferior results of Boneloc-cemented Charnley prostheses (study 1). It also documented that the Exeter prosthesis was inferior using Boneloc, but its results were better than those of the Charnley prosthesis. This can probably be explained by the difference in prosthesis design. The Exeter femoral component has a double tapering section and a polished surface. This design may tolerate bone cement with poor mechanical performance better than the design of the Charnley prosthesis.

The weakness in this study is that we can not control for surgeons' personal cementing techniques. In Norway, it was however normal to use second and third generation cementing techniques, including vacuum mixing during the whole study period. The strength of our study is that the results represent the average surgeon and the performance of implants and cements in a whole nation.

Conclusion

Our studies on prostheses and cements show that, in cemented total hip replacement, the type of cement is more important than the type of femoral prosthesis. Boneloc cement was shown to perform more poorly than high-viscosity cements after only 2 years of follow-up, and the same was shown for the CMW 3 low-viscosity cement after 5 years of observation. Prophylaxis given as a combination of systemic antibiotic and antibiotic-containing cement was associated with fewer revisions due to infection and aseptic loosening.

Acknowledgements. The Norwegian Arthroplasty Register is a team project. We thank our coauthors and the secretaries Adriana Opazo, Kari Strømme, and Inger Skar, the orthopaedic surgeon Professor Lars B. Engesaeter, and the statisticians involved with the register, Professor Stein Emil Vollset and Stein Atle Lie. We are also grateful to the Norwegian orthopaedic surgeons who report their cases to the registry.

References

1. Cox DR (1972) Regression models and life tables. J Royal Stat Soc 34:187–220
2. Espehaug B, Havelin LI, Engesaeter LB, Vollset SE, Langeland N (1995) Early revision among 12,179 hip prostheses. A comparison of 10 different prosthesis brands reported to the Norwegian Arthroplasty Register, 1987–1993. Acta Orthop Scand 66:487–493
3. Espehaug B, Engesaeter LB, Vollset SE, Havelin LI, Langeland N (1997) Antibiotic prophylaxis in total hip arthroplasty. Review of 10,905 primary cemented total hip replacements reported to the Norwegian Arthroplasty Register, 1987–1995. J Bone Joint Surg Br 79B:590–595
4. Furnes O, Lie SA, Havelin LI, Vollset SE, Engesaeter LB (1997) Exeter and Charnley arthroplasties with Boneloc or high viscosity cement. Comparison of 1127 arthroplasties followed for 5 years in the Norwegian Arthroplasty Register. Acta Orthop Scand 68:515–520
5. Havelin LI, Espehaug B, Vollset SE, Engesaeter LB, Langeland N (1993) The Norwegian Arthroplasty Register. A survey of 17,444 total hip replacements. Acta Orthop Scand 64:245–251
6. Havelin LI, Espehaug B, Vollset SB, Engesaeter LB (1994) Early failures among 14,009 cemented and 1,326 uncemented prostheses for primary coxarthrosis. The Norwegian Arthroplasty Register, 1987–1992. Acta Orthop Scand 65:1–6
7. Havelin, LI, Espehaug, B, Vollset, SE, Engesaeter LB (1995) The effect of the type of cement on early revision of Charnley total hip prostheses. A review of 8,579 primary arthroplasties from the Norwegian Arthroplasty Register. J Bone Joint Surg Am 77A: 1543–1550
8. Howie DW, Campbell D, McGee M, Cornish BL (1990) Wagner resurfacing hip arthroplasty. The results of one hundred consecutive arthroplasties after eight to ten years. J Bone Joint Surg Am 72(5)A:708–714
9. Josefsson G, Lindberg L, Wiklander B (1981) Systemic antibiotics and gentamicin-containing bone cement in the prophylaxis of postoperative infections in total hip arthroplasty. Clin Orthop 159:194–200
10. Josefsson G, Gudmundsson G, Kolmert L, Wijkström S (1990) Prophylaxis with systemic antibiotics versus gentamicin bone cement in total hip arthroplasty: A five-year survey of 1688 hips. Clin Orthop 2523:173–178
11. Josefsson G, Kolmert L (1993) Prophylaxis with systematic antibiotics versus gentamicin bone cement in total hip arthroplasty: A ten-year survey of 1688 hips. Clin Orthop 292:210–214
12. Kaplan EL, Meier P (1958) Nonparametric estimation from incomplete observations. J Am Stat Assoc 53:457–481
13. Malchau H (1995) On the importance of stepwise introduction of new hip implant technology. Assessment of total hip replacement using clinical evaluation, radiostereometry, digitised radiography and a national registry. Thesis. Gothenburg, Sweden
14. McQueen MM, Hughes SPF, May P, Verity L (1990) Cefuroxime in total joint arthroplasty: Intravenous or in bone cement. J Arthroplasty 5:169–172
15. Nilsson KG, Kärholm J (1996) RSA in the assessment of aseptic loosening. J Bone Joint Surg Br 78B:1–2
16. Sudmann E, Havelin LI, Lunde OD, Rait M (1983) The Charnley versus the Christiansen total hip arthroplasty. Acta Orthop Scand 54:545–552
17. Tanner J, Freij-Larsson C, Kärholm J, Malchau H, Wesslen B (1995) Evaluation of Boneloc. Acta Orthop Scand 66:207–214

Two-Stage Revision of Infected Arthroplasty

G. H. I. M. WALENKAMP

An infected arthroplasty is comparable to osteomyelitis more than septic arthritis. This holds true for the diagnostic approach and especially for treatment. As in osteomyelitis, treatment possibilities in infected arthroplasty are dependent on the duration or acuteness of the infection, stability of the joint and bones, bone stock, and the ability of the patient to withstand the treatments physically and psychologically. In an infected arthroplasty, the following treatments are used, possibly in combination:

1. Local debridement with prosthesis in situ
2. Debridement with extraction of all prosthesis components and all bone cement
3. Reimplantation of the prosthesis
4. Systemic antibiotics
5. Local antibiotic carriers

The choice of treatment is influenced firstly by the acuteness of the infection: is it an early postoperative infection or a late infection?

In early postoperative infections, treatments 1, 4, and 5 are combined, so the prosthesis remains in situ. The infected joint is extensively surgically debrided, and local and systemic antibiotics are applied. When gentamicin polymethylmethacrylate (PMMA) beads are used as local antibiotics, the space for the beads is limited in a total hip prosthesis (THP) to about 120–180 beads and in a total knee revision (TKR) up to 60–120 beads. In the case of gentamicin-impregnated collagen fleeces, the number of fleeces is influenced more by the maximum dose of gentamicin. Exceeding the dose may lead to renal toxicity. In case local antibiotics are used, all wound layers must be closed separately and be watertight to keep the gentamicin in. Drainage should be used as overflow drainage, instead of suction, for 1 day. Beads are removed after 2–3 weeks and, in case of doubt about healing, the debridement and implantation of local antibiotics should be repeated. Early postoperative infection of a prosthesis is a good indication for resorbable carriers because there is limited space for beads, and removal of the carriers is unnecessary.

The systemically administered antibiotics must be applied in high doses for 3–4 weeks intravenously. Depending on clinical healing and improving laboratory parameters, the oral treatment that follows must be given for up to 3–6 months postoperatively. The exact period cannot be given, but the erythrocyte sedimentation rate (ESR) should remain normalized for a few weeks.

This early postoperative treatment with *corpus alienum* in situ is based on the assumption that the infection is limited to the soft tissues of the operated joint and its wound hematoma and has not yet reached the bone-cement interface. The sooner such treatment is performed in the early postoperative phase the more successful it can be (Fr. *"infection précoce, reprise précoce"*). This should be no later than 3–4 weeks after the primary operation. Healing of the infection is possible in more than 50% of cases if the treatment is early and surgically as well as medically aggressive.

If the infection is not limited to inner wound surfaces but also appears at the deeper prosthesis or cement parts, then the treatment will fail. This may become evident in the beginning of treatment in virulent infections and in patients with a low immune capacity. In other patients, failure of the healing may become apparent after a few months of oral antibiotic treatment: the ESR does not decrease further and the joint remains painful. Also, a period of years of uncertainty may start during which the infection remains low-grade. However, exacerbation will usually occur sooner or later, and in these cases there is the risk of severe sepsis, especially in rheumatoid patients.

In late infections, the prosthesis must always be extracted (treatments 2, 4, and 5) and the infected bone bed and soft tissues debrided, because the infection is always present immediately around the prosthesis itself. Preoperative investigations are unable to give reliable information about which parts of a prosthesis are involved in the infection. Therefore, all components of the prosthesis must be removed as well as all pieces of cement. Antibiotics should be given systemically and the space left by removal of the prosthesis is filled with antibiotic-loaded carriers. As in early infections, removal or exchange of the gentamicin beads after 2 weeks is the most practical treatment. Leaving them in situ longer makes no sense when healing is not appropriate as shown by a decrease in the local antibiotic concentration, and a new debridement is necessary. The 2-week treatment schedule facilitates planning. The disadvantage is that it may be difficult to decide in such a short period of 2 weeks whether healing is appropriate. In some cases, it may therefore be helpful to wait 3 or 4 weeks before reintervention. One should not wait longer because by that time the beads may be fixed by granulation tissue and difficult to remove. Also, the increased soft tissue scarring may cause difficulties in reoperation.

The use of local antibiotic carriers has proven to create very high local antibiotic concentrations without systemic toxic side effects. With gentamicin PMMA beads, a local antibiotic concentration can be achieved of several hundred µg/ml of gentamicin. This is sufficient for most bacteria and moderately resistant germs. However, bacteriologists must estimate the minimal inhibitory concentration (MIC) of the germs instead of the normal characterization (sensitive, intermediate, or resistant) based on systemic treatment. Gentamicin resistance will be too high in *Streptococcus faecalis* and methicillin-resistant *Staphylococci epidermis* (MRSE) and multiresistent *Staphylococcus aureus* (MRSA).

In these cases, other solutions must found, such as the use of (1) no local antibiotics – open wound treatment or a suction drainage system or (2) other antibiotics in the bone cement, e.g., vancomycin or clindamycin. One should be aware that not all antibiotics will be released sufficiently after admixture to PMMA, and some antibiotics are not available as sterile powders to be mixed to the PMMA powder.

Resorbable carriers are also available but mostly still experimentally. At present, two kinds of factory-made gentamicin-PMMA collagen are available in Europe, Garacol® (Essex, Munich, Germany) and Septocoll® (Merck Bio-material GmbH, Darmstadt, Germany). These products create higher local gentamicin concentrations, sometimes up to 1000 µg/ml, and this may be helpful against resistant germs. The higher concentrations, however, also have resulted in more side effects (such as renal dysfunction) when too many fleeces were implanted. Septocoll® has a hydrophobe gentamicin component which results in more prolonged release of the gentamicin, thereby displaying one of the pharmacokinetic properties of gentamicin beads.

Spacers are increasingly used in revision of infected arthroplasties. They are supposed to maintain space between bones better than beads and to release antibiotics as well. They can remain in the joint for weeks or even months and should allow movement and, in hips and shoulders, sometimes even weight-bearing.

These may be helpful when a longer waiting period is needed between treatment of the infection and reimplantation of the prosthesis, more so in the case of TKP than in THP. In TKP, the choice between reimplantation or arthrodesis can be postponed for some time with the help of such a spacer. In THP this is not necessary: reimplantation in a Girdlestone hip resection is not very difficult. Weight-bearing with a spacer may cause bone destruction and spacers may dislocate.

An important disadvantage of spacers may be their limited capacity to release antibiotics. This is a surface phenomenon, and the surface area of spacers is much lower than that of beads, so the release of antibiotics will be, too.

Reimplantation of a prosthesis should be considered taking several aspects into account:

1. Is healing appropriate?
2. Is the bone stock sufficient for fixation of the prosthesis?
3. How virulent was the causative germ and how good the immune capacity of the host?
4. Can the patient stand the revision and treatment of an infected reim-planted prosthesis?
5. Will the function be sufficiently better after reimplantation compared with a Girdlestone operation or arthrodesis?

The reimplantation of the prosthesis can be done in THP as (1) short-term reimplantation – after 2–4 weeks, immediately after the local antibiotic therapy, when the beads or spacers are removed – or (2) long-term reimplantation – after 6–12 months when, after the systemic (oral) antibiotic treatment healing seems appropriate and when the ESR remains low and no infection symptoms are evident. In severe infections with virulent germs and/or low immune capacity, long-term revision is safer. Some patients also need these months to consider the risk of reimplantation. Especially patients with calcification around a Girdlestone hip may have very stable hips with good walking capacity, and they often refrain from reimplantation despite their limited hip flexion.

In TKP, a pseudarthrosis can bear weight with an orthosis, but the instability will mostly cause problems. In knees, the choice between reimplantation and arthrodesis has to be made earlier and, if long-term treatment is not possible, spacers should be used.

VI Osteolysis

Osteolysis Induced by Radio-Opaque Agents

AFSIE SABOKBAR, NICHOLAS A. ATHANASOU, DAVID W. MURRAY

Abstract. In the fibrous membrane surrounding an aseptically loose cemented implant, a heavy infiltrate of foreign body macrophages is commonly seen in response to particles of polymethylmethacrylate (PMMA) bone cement and other biomaterials. We have previously shown that monocytes and macrophages responding to bone cement particles are capable of differentiating into osteoclastic cells that resorb bone. To determine whether radio-opaque additives [barium sulphate ($BaSO_4$) and zirconium dioxide (ZrO_2)] influence this process, particles of PMMA, with or without these radio-opaque agents, were added to mouse monocytes and co-cultured with osteoblast-like cells on bone slices. Osteoclast differentiation was assessed by determining the expression of the osteoclast-associated enzyme tartrate-resistant acid phosphatase (TRAP) and lacunar bone resorption. The addition of PMMA alone to these co-cultures caused no increase in TRAP expression or bone resorption relative to control co-cultures (i.e. no added particles). However, adding PMMA particles containing $BaSO_4$ or ZrO_2 caused an increase in TRAP expression and a highly significant increase in bone resorption. Particles containing $BaSO_4$ were associated with 50% more bone resorption than particles containing ZrO_2. These results suggest that radio-opaque agents in bone cement may contribute to the pathological bone resorption of aseptic loosening by enhancing macrophage-osteoclast differentiation, and that PMMA containing $BaSO_4$ is likely to be associated with more osteolysis than PMMA containing ZrO_2.

Introduction

Aseptic loosening is the major long-term complication of total joint replacements. In the fibrous pseudomembrane surrounding a loose-cemented implant there is a heavy foreign body macrophage and macrophage polykaryon response to polymethylmethacrylate (PMMA) and other implant biomaterial wear particles (Goldring et al. 1983, 1986; Maguire 1987; Goodman et al. 1989; Willert et al. 1990). This foreign body response to biomaterials contributes to the osteolysis of loosening either through particle activation of macrophages to release inflammatory mediators which stimulate resident osteoclasts to resorb bone (Murray and Rushton 1990; Amstutz et al. 1992;

Jiranek et al. 1993; Chiba et al. 1994; Harris 1994) or by differentiation of the particle-associated macrophages into bone-resorbing osteoclasts (Quinn et al. 1992; Sabokbar et al. 1997, 1998).

Contrast agents, notably barium sulphate ($BaSO_4$) and zirconium dioxide (ZrO_2) are commonly added to the bone cement in order to confer radiopacity and thus aid in the X-ray assessment of the implants. The addition of radio-opaque agents to PMMA is, however, not achieved without altering the properties of the bone cement. Although changes in the mechanical strength of the bone cement may be insignificant (Chan and Ahmed 1991), radio-opaque agents are harder than a metallic femoral head, and if they enter the joint space, may cause third-body wear, resulting in damage to the metal articulating surface and, as a consequence, a marked increase in the production of polyethylene wear debris (Issac et al. 1987; Caravia et al. 1990). In addition, there is evidence that these agents evoke a significant pathological response in the surrounding tissue. $BaSO_4$ injected intradermally into experimental animals is known to cause a foreign body inflammatory reaction (Adams 1976); barium has also been shown to intensify the release of inflammatory mediators in response to PMMA particles (Lazarus et al. 1994). Very few reports are available with regards to ZrO_2, although the development of epithelioid granulomas after the injection of elemental zirconium has been reported (Adams 1976).

We have recently shown that macrophages responding to PMMA (which contained $BaSO_4$) (Quinn et al. 1992; Sabokbar et al. 1997, 1998) and other implant biomaterial particles (Pandey et al. 1996) are able to differentiate into osteoclastic cells capable of resorbing bone. For this to occur it is essential that the macrophages are cultured with osteoblast-like cells. The effect of additives in bone cement, such as $BaSO_4$ or ZrO_2, on this process of macrophage-osteoclast differentiation is not known. In this study that has previously been described by Sabokbar et al. (1997), we have determined whether these radio-opaque agents influence this process by adding PMMA particles, with and without the above radio-opaque agents, to monocytes cultured on bone slices with osteoblast-like cells. Osteoclast differentiation was assessed by the expression of osteoclast markers. The bone resorption was quantified by counting the number of pits formed on the surface of the bone slices.

Material and Methods

PMMA Particles

Bone cement was prepared according to the manufacturers' instructions. PMMA alone and PMMA with 9.2% $BaSO_4$ were provided by CMW (Depuy, UK), and PMMA with 15.6% ZrO_2 was provided by Palacos (Schering-Plough, UK). The bone cement was crushed using a steel-mortar pestle and then a Tema Micromill (Siebtechnik, Germany). Size distribution was determined by scanning electron microscopy. This demonstrated that there was a wide range of particle sizes and that the majority (>90%) of the particles were between 1 and 10 μm in diameter. The particles were then weighed, suspended in culture medium, and sonicated for 10 min before being added to culture wells at a concentration of 10 μg/ml.

Materials

For cell culture, alpha minimal essential medium (MEM) was supplemented with 100 IU/ml penicillin, 10 μg/ml streptomycin and 10 mmol L-glutamine and 10% foetal calf serum (FCS) (Gibco, UK). The cloned hormone-responsive osteoblast-like UMR-106 rat cell line, originally derived from a rat osteosarcoma, was generously provided by Professor T.J. Martin (Melbourne, Australia). All incubations were carried out at 37 °C in 5% CO_2.

Isolation of Murine Monocytes

After heart puncture of MF1 female mice, whole blood was layered over Ficoll-Hypaque (Amersham Pharmacia, UK), and centrifuged (693 *g*) for 20 min. The cells at the interface layer were removed and centrifuged at 300 *g* for 10 min, then resuspended in MEM/FCS. The number of live mononuclear cells in the suspension was determined using a haemocytometer.

Preparation of Co-cultures on Human Bone Slices and Coverslips

Monocyte cultures were set up on sterile 6-mm glass coverslips and on human femoral cortical bone slices (10 mm^2) as previously described (Udagawa et al. 1990; Quinn et al. 1992). UMR-106 cells were seeded onto bone slices and coverslips, which had been placed in 7-mm wells of a 96-well tissue culture plate, at a final concentration of $1{\times}10^4$ cells per well and incubated for 24 h at 37 °C; $1{\times}10^5$ monocytes were then added to each well. Control monocyte cultures were also set up on bone slices and coverslips in the absence of UMR-106 cells.

After 2 h of incubation, the bone slices and coverslips were transferred to 17-mm wells containing 1 ml MEM/FCS with $1{\times}10^{-7}$ M 1,25 dihydroxy vitamin D_3 [1,25$(OH)_2D_3$] (Solvay Duphar, Netherlands) and $1{\times}10^{-8}$ M hydrocortisone (Sigma Chemicals, UK). At this point 10 μg/ml of the various PMMA particles (with and without $BaSO_4$ or ZrO_2) were added to the wells. As controls, additional wells were also set up where no particles were added. The cultures were maintained for 7 and 14 days, with the media containing all the factors being replenished every 3 days.

Histochemical Characterisation of Cultured Cells

After 7 days, using a kit from Sigma Chemicals (UK), coverslips were stained for TRAP which is an osteoclast-associated enzyme (Minkin 1982).

Scanning Electron Microscopy Examination of Bone Slices to Determine Resorption Pit Formation

After 14 days in culture, bone slices were rinsed vigorously in distilled water and immersed in 0.25 M NH_4OH for 24 h to remove the cells and cell debris from the bone surface. After alcohol dehydration, the bone slices were mounted onto aluminium stubs (Abbot Laboratories, UK), sputter-coated with gold, and examined using a Philips SEM 505 scanning electron microscope.

Assessment of Bone Resorption and Statistical Analysis

The results were expressed as the number of bone resorption pits per bone slice, which has been shown to provide a good correlation with the total surface area of bone resorbed (Chambers et al. 1984) as the volume and area of individual resorption pits is known to fall within a defined range (Athanasou et al. 1984). In each experiment, four bone slices were used for each individual treatment (i.e. control, PMMA alone, $PMMA+BaSO_4$, and $PMMA+ZrO_2$). Each experiment was carried out six times. Two separate statistical analyses were carried out. In the first analysis, the average number of pits in each experiment for each treatment was determined (Table 1), and compared using a paired Student's t test ($n=6$). In the second analysis, the results from each bone slice were compared using two-way analysis of variance (Sokal and Rohlf 1981). These analyses give greater insight into the data.

Results

Histochemical Characterisation of Isolated and Cultured Cells

Giemsa-staining of monocyte cultures incubated in the presence of PMMA particles (±radio-opaque agents) revealed that mononuclear cells were capable of phagocytosing these particles; cells contained numerous clear, small, polarisable PMMA particles in the cytoplasm (Fig. 1).

After 7 days in culture with UMR-106 cells, and in the presence of $1,25(OH)_2D_3$, clusters of TRAP[+] cells were noted in control and PMMA-containing co-cultures (Fig. 2). Many more TRAP[+] cells and cell clusters were noted in the co-cultures to which $PMMA+BaSO_4$ and $PMMA+ZrO_2$ had been added.

Table 1. The mean number of resorption pits formed in UMR-106-monocyte co-cultures after 14 days incubation in the presence or absence of PMMA particles (with and without radio-opaque agents). For each experiment, the mean and the standard deviation (SD) of the number of pits formed on four bone slices are given. The experiments were repeated six times. The final column shows the mean and SD values for all six experiments

Treatment	Expt. 1 mean (SD)	Expt. 2 mean (SD)	Expt. 3 mean (SD)	Expt. 4 mean (SD)	Expt. 5 mean (SD)	Expt. 6 mean (SD)	Total mean±SD
Control (no added particles)	35.2 (8.7)	29.7 (4.0)	23.7 (7.2)	25 (11.2)	26.7 (11.2)	27.5 (11.7)	28±9.2
PMMA alone	24.5 (5.7)	17.5 (7.3)	17.5 (5.4)	24.8 (12.4)	27.8 (9.4)	26.8 (8.9)	23.1±8.6
PMMA+BaSO$_4$	90.2 (19.4)	93.5 (12.9)	72.7 (22.9)	120.2 (32.7)	147 (34.2)	125 (22.8)	108.1±33.9
PMMA+ZrO$_2$	108.7 (22.7)	41.5 (16.2)	62.5 (19.1)	85.5 (14.4)	97.5 (7.5)	65 (7.4)	76.8±27.7

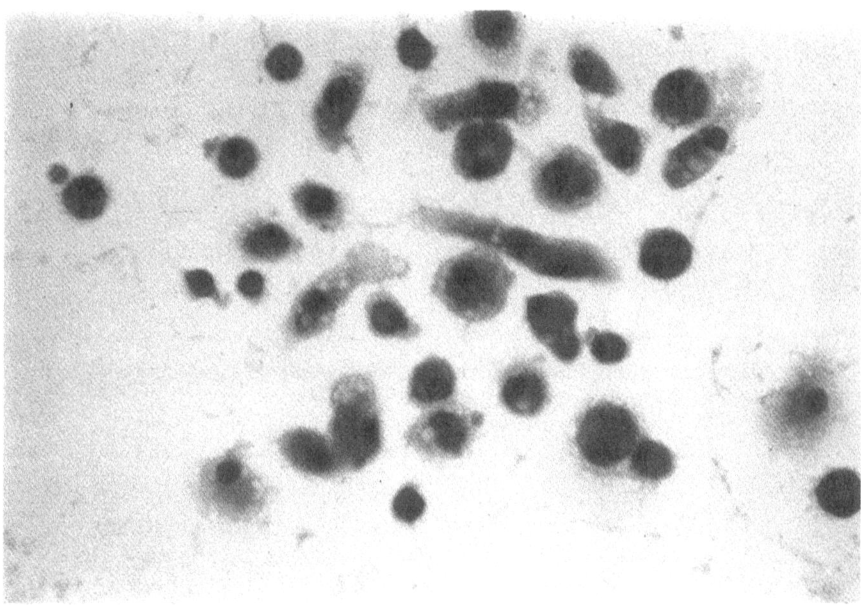

Fig. 1. 24 hour culture of isolated monocytes to which PMMA + BaSO$_4$ particles had been added, showing numerous clear vacuoles containing radio-opaque particles in the cell cytoplasm. (Giemsa ×400, half polarised)

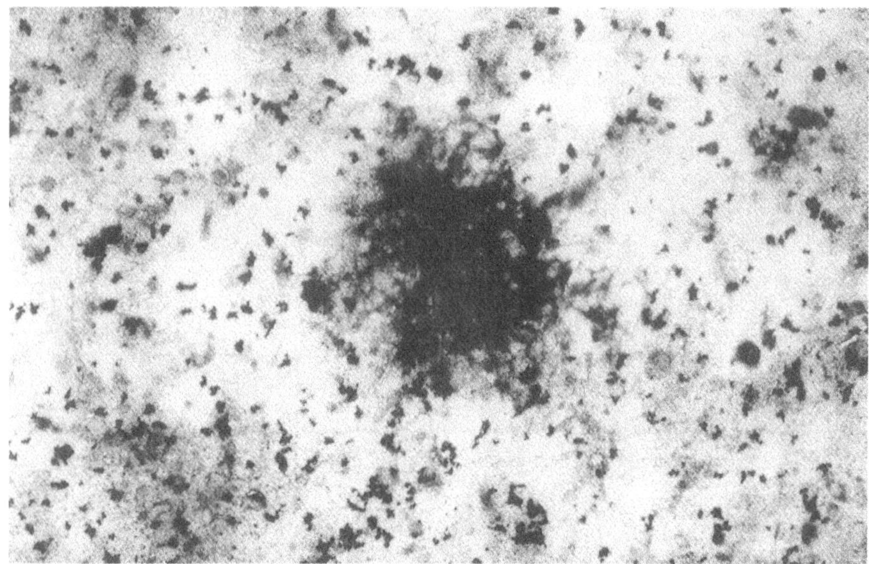

Fig. 2. Histochemical staining of co-cultures of UMR 106 cells and monocytes to which PMMA + BaSO$_4$ had been added. This shows a large cluster of TRAP positive cells ($\times$100)

In the absence of UMR-106 or 1,25(OH)$_2$D$_3$, TRAP$^+$ cell clusters were not seen in 7 day control or PMMA-containing monocyte cultures, indicating that osteoclast differentiation had not occurred.

Lacunar Bone Resorption Characteristics of Isolated and Cultured Cells: The Effect of Radio-Opaque Agents

After 14 days incubation, co-cultures of macrophage and UMR-106 cells, to which PMMA alone had been added, showed no significant increase in resorption pit formation relative to control co-cultures (i.e. those to which no PMMA particles had been added) (Table 1, Fig. 3). However, in co-cultures containing either PMMA+BaSO$_4$ or PMMA+ZrO$_2$, there was a highly significant increase in bone resorption relative to the same control ($p<0.0001$ and $p<0.001$, respectively, $n=6$, t test). Similarly, significantly more bone resorption was seen in those co-cultures to which PMMA+BaSO$_4$ and PMMA+ZrO$_2$ particles had been added relative to the co-cultures containing PMMA particles alone (i.e. PMMA without the radio-opaque agents) ($p<0.0001$ and $p<0.002$, $n=6$, t test).

In addition, PMMA+BaSO$_4$ was found to cause almost 50% more bone resorption than PMMA+ZrO$_2$. This difference only just reached significance ($p=0.05$, $n=6$) when the mean results were compared using a paired t test. However, comparing these results using a two-way analysis of variance, where data from each bone slice in all six experiments are considered, it

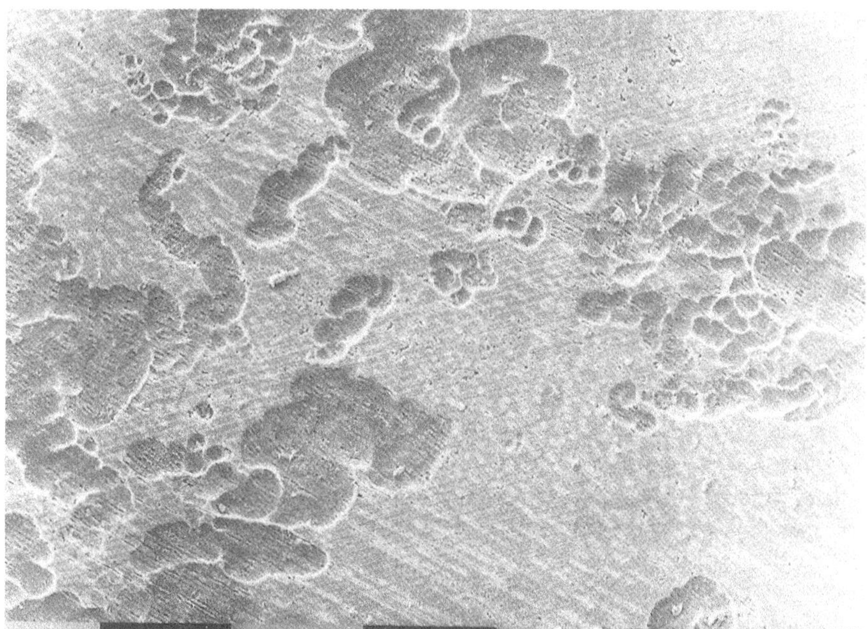

Fig. 3. SEM photomicrograph of human bone slice on which a co-culture of UMR-106 cells and monocytes, to which $PMMA + ZrO_2$ had been added, were incubated for 14 days. This shows extensive lacunar bone resorption with the formation of numerous resorption pits (Grey Bar = 100 μm)

could be seen that there were highly significant differences between each treatment. In particular, it confirmed that $PMMA+BaSO_4$ caused more bone resorption than $PMMA+ZrO_2$, and that this difference was highly significant ($p<0.0001$, $n=24$). It also confirmed that PMMA alone did not cause more bone resorption than the control.

Discussion

The fibrous pseudomembrane surrounding a loose cemented arthroplasty component commonly contains a heavy macrophage and macrophage poly-karyon response to small and large fragments of PMMA cement. Two agents, $BaSO_4$ and ZrO_2, are often incorporated into the PMMA cement in order to render it radio-opaque. Histologically, these are evident as small polarisable granules present on the surface of PMMA spheres (Willert et al. 1974; Mirra et al. 1976; Revell 1982; Forest et al. 1991; Bos et al. 1995). Autopsy studies have shown that both $BaSO_4$ and ZrO_2 are present in the methacrylate implant bed (Willert et al. 1974; Huo et al. 1992) and high levels of $BaSO_4$ (Betts et al. 1990) and ZrO_2 (Bos et al. 1990; Keen et al. 1992) have been found in the periprosthetic tissues from failed implants.

We have previously shown that macrophages responding to bone cement particles are capable of differentiating into osteoclastic cells that cause lacunar bone resorption when cultured in the presence of osteoblast-like cells and $1,25(OH)_2D_3$ (Quinn et al. 1992; Sabokbar et al. 1997, 1998). In this study, we have shown that particles of PMMA containing the radio-opaque additives $BaSO_4$ and ZrO_2 greatly enhance this process of macrophage-osteoclast differentiation as compared to PMMA particles alone. This was seen not only as an increase in expression of the osteoclast-associated enzyme TRAP, but also, correspondingly, as a highly significant increase in the extent of lacunar bone resorption. Moreover, this study has shown that $PMMA+BaSO_4$ increases lacunar resorption pit formation by almost 50% compared with $PMMA+ZrO_2$. This is despite the fact that more ZrO_2 than $BaSO_4$ was present in the bone cements used in this study (i.e. 15.6% compared to 9.2%).

Figure 4 schematically represents the cellular mechanism which may be involved in the process of PMMA-induce osteoclast formation. We propose that in the pseudomembrane formed around joint arthroplasties, particle-associated macrophages can differentiate into osteoclastic bone resorbing cells when they are in contact with osteoblast-like cells on the bone surface. It is now known that osteoblasts express a membrane-associated factor known as osteoclast differentiation factor (ODF; also known as TRANCE, OPGL, and RANKL) (Jimi et al. 1998; Lacey et al. 1998) that binds its specific receptor RANK expressed on osteoclast precursors (Nakagawa et al. 1998). Upon the binding of these factors and in the presence of a soluble factor called macrophage colony stimulating factor (M-CSF), which is released by resident and activated osteoblasts (Roodman 1996), bone resorbing osteoclasts can be formed. Another soluble factor released by osteoblasts and stromal cells is osteoprotegerin (OPG). This inhibits the ODF/RANK interaction by binding to ODF and hence inhibits osteoclast formation (Simonet et al. 1997). Therefore, osteoclast formation in periprosthetic tissues can be viewed as a balance between the production of ODF and OPG by stromal cells and inflammatory cells at the bone and implant interface.

In this study we aimed to present the radio-opaque agents to the macrophages in the manner that they occur clinically. Instead of adding radio-opaque agents directly to the cultures, we made up bone cement with radio-opaque additives according to manufacturers' instructions and then crushed it and added the particles to the cultures. Therefore, there are slight differences in the cement associated with the different radio-opaque agents. For example, the cement containing ZrO_2 (Palacos) had a small amount of methacrylate copolymer and chlorophyll, which was not present in the $BaSO_4$-containing cement (CMW). However, the basic constituent of the cements, methylmethacrylate, activators, and antibiotics were the same. The differences between the cements were small and it is highly unlikely that they, rather than the different radio-opaque agent, would account for the large (50%) differences in bone resorption. Furthermore, the CMW cement containing $BaSO_4$ caused more bone resorption than the Palacos cement containing ZrO_2. This suggests that the increased resorption is either caused by $BaSO_4$ or something in the CMW cement. However, the CMW cement with-

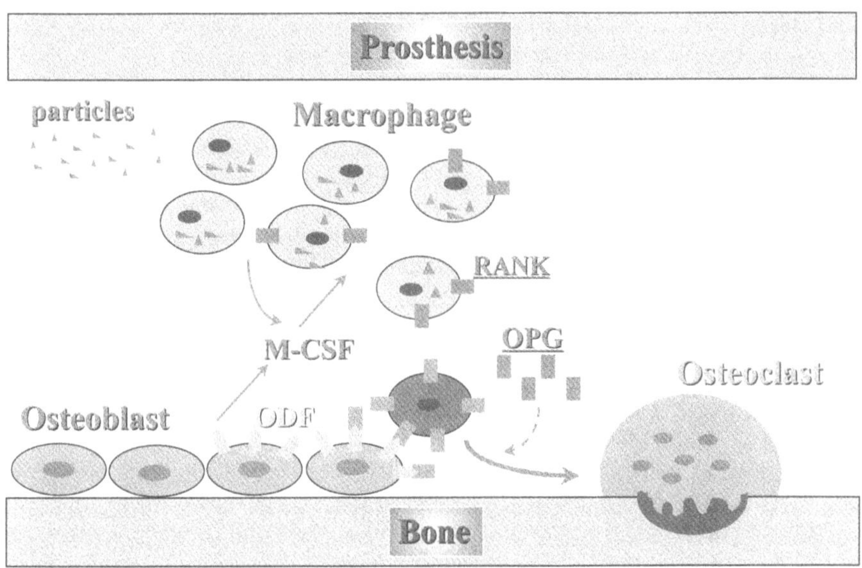

Fig. 4. Schematic presentation of the possible cellular mechanism involved in particle-induced osteolysis

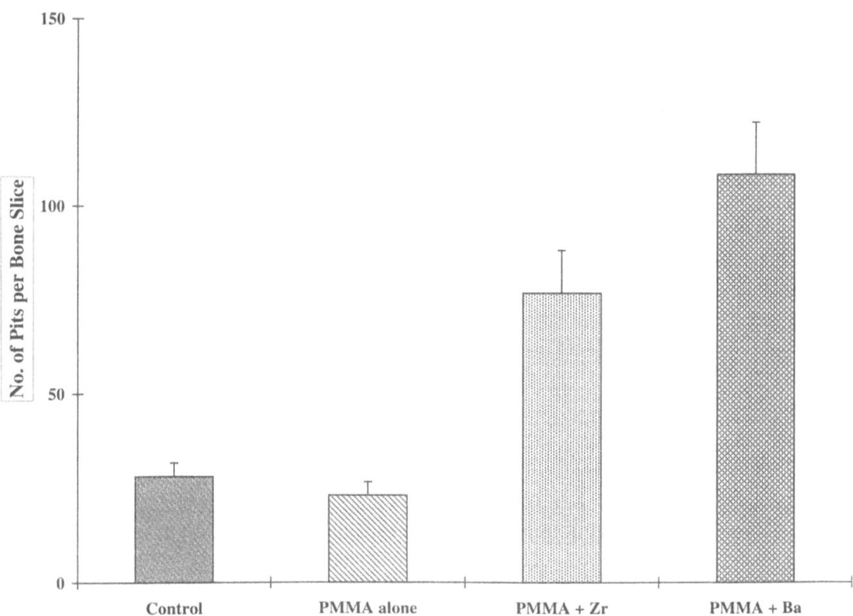

Fig. 5. Mean number of resorption pits (± standard error of the mean) formed per bone slice in culture conditions in which UMR-106/monocyte co-cultures were set up in the presence of (a) no particles, (b) PMMA particles alone, (c) PMMA + BaSO$_4$ (Ba) particles and (d) PMMA + ZrO$_2$ (Zr) particles, for 14 days. For the levels of significance, refer to „Results" section

out $BaSO_4$ caused the same amount of resorption as control, so the differences are almost certainly caused by the radio-opaque agents.

There are remarkably few data on the biological effects of adding $BaSO_4$ or ZrO_2 to PMMA. This is despite the fact that substances such as barium are known to have the capacity to be quite toxic if absorbed. A localised granulomatous reaction to $BaSO_4$ in the bowel wall may rarely follow the use of radio-opaque agents in barium enemas (Sasson 1960; Patros 1994). A granulomatous disease of the lung, barytosis, has also been reported in workers engaged in the barium ore industry (Blum 1962). Moreover, the intradermal injection of $BaSO_4$ into experimental animals is known to evoke an inflammatory granulomatous cellular response (Adams 1976). However, Rae (1977) found no apparent cytotoxic effect when $BaSO_4$ was added to cultured mouse macrophages.

Lazarus et al. (1994), using a rat subcutaneous air pouch model, have shown that compared to PMMA particles alone, the addition of PMMA particles containing $BaSO_4$ to these synovial-lined cavities, significantly enhances the local release of known stimulators of osteoclastic bone resorption such as prostaglandins and tumour necrosis factor, as well as neutral proteases and other inflammatory mediators. The authors also inserted non-weight-bearing plugs of PMMA (with or without $BaSO_4$) in the distal femurs of rats after which each knee was injected with PMMA particulates with and without $BaSO_4$. They found that $PMMA+BaSO_4$ particles caused significantly greater bone resorption than did particulates of PMMA that did not contain additives. In our study, although we cannot exclude the possibility that some of the increase in bone resorption seen in our co-cultures was due to an effect of $BaSO_4$ on the activity of formed osteoclasts, this would appear unlikely, as this increase in bone resorption was associated with an observed increase in the number of cells expressing TRAP in those co-cultures to which particles of PMMA containing radio-opaque agents were added as compared to those containing particles of PMMA alone. This would indicate that a major effect of adding PMMA particles containing $BaSO_4$ or ZrO_2 to monocytes is to increase significantly their differentiation into osteoclasts.

Although, there are numerous in vitro studies which describe possible toxicological and biological effects of PMMA, few of these indicate whether these effects are in response to PMMA alone or to PMMA containing radio-opaque agents or other additives (for review, see Amstutz et al. 1992). Our study shows that compared with the effect of adding PMMA alone, the addition of PMMA particles containing radio-opaque agents to mononuclear phagocytes in vitro produced significantly different results with respect to cell differentiation and function. This would indicate that it is essential for future in vitro (and probably in vivo) studies on bone cement to specify the constituents of the PMMA employed.

Although radio-opaque agents are added to bone cement in order to aid the assessment of implants, they are not essential for this purpose. For example, the most important features of implant loosening, bone resorption, and implant migration can be detected by means of serial X-rays without using radio-opaque bone cement. Therefore, in order to avoid the risk of radio-opaque agents contributing to bone resorption and implant loosening, consideration may be given to using bone cement without radio-opaque additives. However, if radio-opaque agents are felt to be essential for the assessment of an implant, then radio-opaque agents that do not greatly enhance the differentiation of PMMA-associated macrophages into bone resorbing osteoclasts should be employed. Our findings suggest that bone cement containing ZrO_2 is preferable to cement containing $BaSO_4$ in this regard. The osteolytic consequences of radio-opaque agents may also possibly be reduced by decreasing the concentration of these agents in PMMA or by developing new radio-opaque agents that do not increase osteoclast differentiation by biomaterial wear particle-associated macrophages. The in vitro system used in this study should provide a useful model whereby these alternatives can be explored (Fig 5).

References

Adams DO (1976) The granulomatous inflammatory response: a review. Am J Pathol 84: 164–191

Amstutz HC, Campbell P, Kossovsky N, Clarke IC (1992) Mechanism and clinical significance of wear debris-induced osteolysis. Clin Orthop Rel Res 276:7–18

Athanasou NA, Gray A, Revell PA, Fuller K, Cochrane T, Chambers TJ (1984) Stereophotogrammetric observations on bone resorption by isolated osteoclasts. Micron and Microscopica Acta 15:47–53

Betts F, Wright T, Salvati E, Boskey A (1990) Barium content of tissues from revision total hip arthroplasties. Trans Orthop Res Soc 15:457

Blum CK (1962) Radiology of some rarer dust diseases (barytosis, asbestosis and siderosis). Scot Med J 7:478–487

Bos I, Fredebold D, Diebold J, Lohrs U (1995) Tissue reactions to cemented hip sockets. Histologic and morphometric autopsy study of 25 acetabula. Acta Orthop Scand 66(1): 1–8

Bos I, Johannisson R, Lohrs U, Lindner B, Seydel U (1990) Comparative investigations of regional lymph nodes and pseudocapsules after implantation of joint endoprostheses. Pathol Res Pract 186(6):707–716

Caravia L, Dowson D, Fisher J, Jobbins B (1990) The influence of bone and bone cement debris on counterface roughness in sliding wear of ultra high molecular weight polyethylene on stainless steel. Proceedings of Institute of Mechanical Engineering 204:65–70

Chambers TJ, Revell PA, Fuller K, Athanasou NA (1984) Resorption of bone by isolated rabbit osteoclasts. J Cell Science, 66:383–399

Chan KH, Ahmed AM (1991) Polymethylmethacrylate. In: BF Morrey (ed) Joint Replacement Arthroplasty. Churchill Livingstone, London, pp 23–37

Chiba J, Rubash HE, Kangjung Kim, Yuichi Iwaki et al (1994) The characterisation of cytokines in the interface tissue obtained from failed cementless total hip arthroplasties with/without femoral osteolysis. Clin Orthop Rel Res 300:304–312

Forest M, Carlioz A, Vacher Lavenu MC, Postel M, Kerboull M, Tomeno B, Courpied JP (1991) Histological patterns of bone and articular tissues after orthopaedic reconstructive surgery (artificial joint implants). Path Res Prac 187:963–977

Goldring SR, Jasty M, Roelke MS, Rourke CM, Bringhurst FR, Harris WH (1986) Formation of a synovial like membrane at the bone cement interface. Arthritis Rheum 29:836–842

Goldring SR, Schiller AL, Roelke M, Rourke CM, O'Neill DA, Harris WH (1983) The synovial-like membrane at the bone cement interface in loose total hip replacements and its proposed role in bone lysis. J Bone Joint Surg [Am] 65A:386–342

Goodman SB, Chris RC, Chiou SS et al (1989) A clinical, pathological, biochemical study of the membrane surrounding loosened and non loosened total hip arthroplasties. Clin Orthop Rel Res 244:182–187

Harris WH (1994) Osteolysis and particle disease in hip replacement: a review. Acta Orthop Scand 65:113–123

Huo MH, Salvati EA, Liberman JR, Betts F, Basal M (1992) Metallic debris in femoral endo-steolysis in failed cemented total hip arthroplasties. Clin Orthop Rel Res 276:157–168

Issac GH, Atkinson JR, Dowson, D, Kennedy PD, Smith MR (1987) The causes of femoral head roughening in explanted Charnley hip prostheses. Engineering in Medicine 16:167–173

Jimi E, Akiyama S, Tsurukai T, Kobayashi K, Takahashi N, Udagawa N, Shima N, Kinosaki M, Yamaguchi K, Morinaga T, Higashio K, and Suda T (1998) Osteoclast differentiation factor (ODF) induces fusion, survival and activation of osteoclasts. J Bone Miner Res 23:S222

Jiranek WA, Machado M, Jasty M et al (1993) Production of cytokines around loosened cemented acetabular components. J Bone Joint Surg [Am] 75A:863–879

Keen CE, Philip G, Brady K, Spencer JD, Levison DA (1992) Histopathological and micro-analytical study of zirconium dioxide and barium sulphate in bone cement. J Clin Pathol 45:984–989

Lacey DL, Timms E, Tan H-L, Kelley MJ, Dunstan CR, Burgess T, Elliott R, Colombero A, Elliott G, Scully S, Hsu H, Sullivan J, Hawkins N, Davy E, Capparelli C, Eli A, Qian Y-X, Kaufman S, Sarosi I, Shalhoub V, Senaldi G, Guo J, Delaney J, Boyle WJ (1998) Osteopro-tegerin ligand is a cytokine that regulates osteoclast differentiation and activation. Cell 93:165–176

Lazarus MD, Cuckler JM, Schumacher HR, Ducheyne P, Baker DG (1994) Comparison of the inflammatory response to particulate polymethylmethacrylate debris with and with-out barium sulfate. J Orthop Res 12(4):532–541

Maguire JK (1987) Foreign body reaction to polymeric debris following total hip arthro-plasty. Clin Orthop 216:213–223

Minkin C (1982) Bone acid phosphatase-tartrate-resistant acid phosphatase as a marker of osteoclast function. Calcif Tissue Int 34:285–290

Mirra JM, Amstutz HC, Matos M, Gold R (1976) The pathology of the joint tissues and its clinical relevance in prosthesis failure. Clin Orthop Rel Res 117:221–240

Murray DW, Rushton N (1990) Macrophages stimulate bone resorption when they phago-cytose particles. J Bone Joint Surg [Br] 72B:988–992

Nakagawa N, Kinosaki M, Yamaguchi K, Shima N, Yasuda H, Yano K, Morinaga T, and Higashio K (1998) RANK is the essential signaling receptor for osteoclast differentiation factor in osteoclastogenesis. Biochem Biophys Res Commun 253:395–400

Pandey R, Quinn J, Joyner C, Murray DW, Triffitt JT, Athanasou NA (1996) Arthroplasty im-plant biomaterial-associated macrophages differentiate into lacunar bone-resorbing cells. Ann Rheum Dis 55(6):388–395

Patros RE (1994) Non neoplastic intestinal diseases. In: Sternbers SS, (ed) Diagnostic surgi-cal pathology, 2nd ed, Raven Press, NY, pp 1358

Quinn JM, Joyner C, Triffitt JT, Athanasou N (1992) PMMA-induced inflammatory macro-phages resorb bone. J Bone Joint Surg [Br] 74B:652–658

Rae T (1977) Tolerance of mouse macrophages in vitro to barium sulphate used in ortho-paedic bone cement J Biomed Mat Res 11:839–846

Revell PA (1982) Tissue reactions to joint prostheses and the products of wear and corro-sion. In: Berry CL (ed) Bone and Joint Disease, Current Topics in Pathology 17. Springer, Berlin, pp 37–101

Roodman, G.D (1996) Advances in bone biology: the osteoclast. Endocrine Rev 17:308–332

Sabokbar A, Fujikawa Y, Brett J, Murray DW, Athanasou NA (1997) Increased osteoclastic differentiation by polymethylmethacrylate wear particle-associated macrophages: Inhibi-tion by interleukin-4 and leukaemia inhibitory factor. Acta Orthop Scand 67(6):593–598

Sabokbar A, Pandey R, Quinn J, Athanasou NA (1998) Osteoclastic differentiation by mono-nuclear phagocytes containing biomaterial particles. Arch Orthop Trauma Surg 184:31–36

Sasson L (1960) Entrace of barium into intestinal glands during barium enema. J Am Med Assoc 173:343–345

Simonet WS, Lacey DL, Dunstan CR, Kelley M, Chang MS, Luthy R, Nguyen HQ, Wooden S, Bennett L, Boone T, Shimamoto G, DeRose M, Elliott R, Colombero A, Tan HL, Trail G, Sullivan J, Davy E, Bucay N, Renshaw-Gegg L, Hughes TM, Hill D, Pattison W, Camp-bell P, Boyle WJ (1997) Osteoprotegerin: a novel secreted protein involved in the regula-tion of bone density. Cell 89:309–319

Sokal RP, Rohlf FJ (1981) Biometry. 2nd ed, WH Freeman, NY, pp 321–367

Udagawa N, Takahashi N, Akatsu T et al (1974) Origin of osteoclasts: Mature monocytes and macrophages are capable of differentiating into osteoclasts under a suitable micro-environment prepared by bone marrow-derived stromal cells (1990) Proc Natl Acad Sci USA 87:7260–7264

Willert HG, Bertran H, Buchhorn GH (1990) Osteolysis in alloarthroplasty of the hip: The role of bone cement fragmentation. Clin Orthop Rel Res 258:108–111
Willert HG, Ludwig J, Semlitsch M (1974) Reaction of bone to methacrylate after hip arthroplasty. A long term gross, light microscopic and scanning electron microscopic study. J Bone Joint Surg [Am] 56A(7):1368–1382

Wear and Osteolyses

GOTTFRIED H. BUCHHORN, HANS-GEORG WILLERT

Introduction

During the operative procedure, not only the remainders of articular carti-lage but also subcortical lamellae, spongious bone, and cortical structures are reamed or sawn off. In the case of a total hip joint replacement, the femoral head and parts of the femoral neck are totally removed and the intertrochanteric spongious bone is partially removed. The medullary canal is reamed to provide space for the anchoring device. In areas of spongious bone the self-supporting interconnection is broken up and the bone marrow is exposed.

A completely new interface between implant and bone is built up during the process of "healing in" which follows the implantation of the endopros-thesis. This healing reaction of the implant bed closely resembles the process of fracture healing in the course of which destroyed and necrotic bone and bone marrow are replaced by new bone as in callus formation.

Zones of noncontact between the device (bone cement, polymer, or metal implant) and the anchoring bone are initially filled with blood and detritus that become organized by ingrowing granulation tissue during the process of healing. Later, the granulation tissue is replaced either by fibrous tissue, which may transform into fat- and hematopoietic bone marrow, or by new bone, depending on the biomechanical need and the width of the gap. A so-called permanent implant bed will be formed after the phase of repair. The interface between implant and bone then consists of vital bone as well as of fat marrow and hematopoietic bone marrow. With some biomaterials (e.g., poly-methylmethacrylate), the implants are covered by delicate membranes of connective tissue and giant cells. Direct contact of bone to all polyethylene implant devices is very uncommon. Usually an interconnecting layer of cells or even a layer of fibrous tissue is observed. The composition of the gross tissue structures at the interface is basically the same with cemented and noncemented implants; only multinuclear giant cells are more abundant around bone cement, while they are relatively lacking around noncemented implants [66, 67, 72, 79]. Under optimal conditions, the implants are toler-ated by the biological environment and do not overstress the anchoring bone. Implants do not induce pain as long as they stay firmly fixed to the bone [13].

If the joint capsule has been resected in the course of the surgical procedure, a new capsule is formed around the artificial joint. Its architecture roughly resembles a normal joint capsule with an inner synovial, an intermediate vascular, and an outer fibrous layer.

Remodelling and Adaptation of Bone

It is a long-known fact that in mature bone neither new formation nor resorption occurs separately. Therefore, the continuous process of bone remodelling comprises both new bone formation and bone resorption. Preponderance of either new bone formation or bone resorption will increase or decrease the bone mass [17]. In general, the regulation of the coincidental appearance of osteoblastic and osteoclastic activity has been termed "coupling mechanism" [17].

The implant-carrying bone is subjected to physiologic remodelling like any other bone of the skeleton. After the process of healing, it can be assumed that mass, structure, and orientation of the implant-carrying bone are adjusted to the strain that is applied in the course of loading and motion exerted by the patient [7]. Especially stair climbing and sitting down/standing up as well as acceleration due to more-or-less controlled movements in daily activity or sports result in the application of the resulting load towards a direction eccentric to the rotation axis of the anchoring device. In a balanced situation the resulting strain on the implant's surface and the anchoring tissue should not lead to separation of surfaces or to ruptures and fractures of biological structures.

Loosening of Implants

The biology of the loosening of implants is independent of either cemented or noncemented fixation. Wear, tear, and fatigue of implant materials, durability of implant fixation, and stress-shielding of the implant-bearing bone remain unsolved but important problems of total hip replacements. Septic and aseptic loosening have to be differentiated. Septic loosening is caused by bacteria, whereas aseptic loosening is caused by mechanical instability, wear, degradation, corrosion products of implant materials, and hyperergic reactions. Both forms of loosening are caused by inflammatory and granulomatous tissue reactions that induce loss of bone and thus failure of the fixation between implant and bone.

Mechanical loosening at the interface between implant and bone results from loss of the bony anchors mainly due to nonphysiologic bone resorption known as osteolysis. This may occur in the form of diffuse osteolyses throughout the interface or in the form of localized osteolyses in circumscribed areas. There are many reasons for osteolysis, but the processes lead-

ing to bone resorption are always related to the proliferation of a granulomatous tissue adjacent to the implant.

Wear

Wherever surfaces move against each other, either desired as in the case of
articulations or undesired as in the case of failed anchorage, destruction of
the surfaces occurs. The actual loss of material releases wear particles. The
biological significance of the particle size of metal or polyethylene wear became a significant part of the discussion on the contribution of wear to loosening. The majority wear particles (especially those of polyethylene) have
been found to be in the submicron range [11, 25, 44, 45].

As there is always destruction of all articulating surfaces we have to consider loss of material even if it is invisible to our eye. This means that in the
articulation of metal/polyethylene not only polyethylene particles but also
small amounts of metal are released. The release of microscopically invisible
metal wear (either particulate or ions) falls under the aspects of metal corrosion and repassivation; these aspects, however, shall not be discussed here.

The kind, number, and size of liberated wear particles depends on the
abrasion resistance and the surface characteristics of the materials involved
and the pressure acting on the moving surfaces. The resistance of a material
to three-body abrasion by hard particulates is directly proportional to the
hardness of the subjected surfaces [16]. In general, polymers like polyethylene or polymethylmethacrylate (PMMA) wear out more extensively, while
other materials, like metal or ceramic, wear out less [60–62, 64, 68, 77, 78].

Wear from Articulating Surfaces

Particles from the articulating surfaces in general are released into the joint
cavity. They originate from materials such as polymer (nowadays mostly
polyethylene), metal alloys, or ceramic (Fig. 1).

Wear from Anchoring Surfaces

Wear products from anchoring surfaces reach both the implant/bone-inter-
face and the joint cavity from the onset of abrasion. This presupposes undesired motion between the surfaces involved such as PMMA, metal alloys, and
possibly, hydroxyapatite or ceramic coating [8, 34, 69]. The abrasive wear has
a polishing effect on the surfaces where the movement occurs (Fig. 1).

a) articulating surfaces 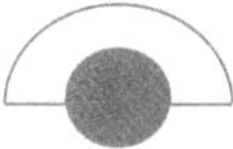

b) anchoring devices 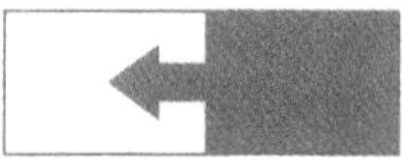

c) component junctions 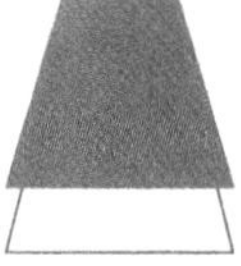

Fig. 1. Sources of particle release: (a) articulating surfaces (area contact, cylinders, ball-bearings), (b) anchoring devices (planes, macro-, microstructures), (c) component junctions (form fit, taper locks, screw and nut)

Wear from Cone Taper Locks

Wear or corrosion products from cone taper locks, though a rare mode of failure, are released into the joint cavity. Multi-component fixation devices, mostly used in revision or tumor surgery may also release wear or corrosion products directly into areas of anchoring bone or encompassing soft tissues (Fig. 1).

Wear particles from the cone taper locks come from metal alloys or ceramic. Corrosion has been reported from combinations of titanium alloy (neck) and CoCr alloy (head) [14, 15]. But corrosion and wear can only develop if fretting between the head and the tapered neck occurs [33]. Loosening of the ceramic head from the metal taper gives rise to abrasive wear from the metal taper, and sometimes, to a very large extent, also from the ceramic head [47].

Characterization of Wear Products

Wear particles from different materials are characterized by their features: amount, size distribution, shape, surface characteristics, and chemical composition.

In this chapter, features of wear products most often observed in routine histology will be summarized. They have been described in detail elsewhere [63, 70, 73].

Metal wear particles originate from stainless steel, CoCrMo- and CoNiCr-alloys, cpTi, and Ti-alloys. Their sizes range mostly from 1 μm or less up to 5 μm (submicron dimensions have often been observed with scanning electron microscopy and transmission electron microscopy). The shape may be described as grains with sharp edges and points. Surfaces appear to be rough.

The size of ultrahigh molecular weight polyethylene (UHMWPE) wear particles are mostly in the range of 1 µm or less up to 50 µm. There are chips and fragments up to several millimeters in size (wear in the submicron size range was isolated with tissue digestion). The shape can be described as elongated, flat grains with points. The surfaces are undulated, sometimes covered with small fibrils.

In light microscopy, PMMA bone-cement wear particles can only be seen in frozen sections; the sizes are up to 50 µm and they appear as polygonal grains. Larger particles can clearly be identified as fragments of pearls with or without attachment of matrix PMMA; these often have diameters up to 200 µm. Further on there are large conglomerates of pearls with or without binding PMMA matrix. The surfaces of the larger fragments are characterized by the pearl structures.

Contrast media, either ZrO_2 or $BaSO_4$, are contained within the PMMA matrix. They are released, however, in case of fragmentation of the composite material and abrasion against bone, metal, and PMMA itself. These grains are then released and their original grain size becomes obvious – ZrO_2, 8 µm (agglomerates up to 50 µm), and $BaSO_4$, 2 µm (agglomerates up to 100 µm). The shape of the grains is predominantly round with some flat edges.

In a few cases we also observed Ti-alloy corrosion products, i.e., TiO_2 in the crystalline forms of anatase and rutile. The size of the grains ranged at around 2 µm; plates skip off from the surfaces and measure up to 150 µm. The shape of the grains is polygonal, the flakes look like scales, and thick plates consist of slate-like layers.

Our description of the relationship of wear and osteolyses is based on macroscopic and microscopic analyses of retrieved tissues and devices from revision cases. For the description of the cellular reactions the following terms will be used:

Monocyte is a general term for a cell with only one nucleus that does not characterize its task or function. A *progenitor* cell is a pluripotent cell with one nucleus, which may enter tissues from the blood stream (hematopoietic) or originate from fibrous tissues (desmal). Depending on regulatory mechanisms, these nondifferentiated cells undergo changes to become specialized cells (e.g., macrophages, osteoclasts).

The *osteoblast* and the *osteoclast* are part of a system to regulate the modelling of bone. Resting osteoblasts cover the surfaces of regular bone and form an endosteal layer between the marrow and bone. Activated osteoblasts form layers of new bone, not yet mineralized (osteoid) (cf. Fig. 8).

The osteoclast is the opponent to the osteoblast as it resorbs bone substance. It is mostly a multinuclear cell and originates from the fusion of mononuclear osteoclast progenitor cells. Whereas the osteoblast appears to be a more permanent cell, the osteoclast is a cell with a short lifespan. Compared to osteoblasts, the osteoclasts appear in smaller numbers. The osteocytes are the cells of the bone tissue, enclosed within the *osteocyte* lacunae.

Monocytes rest in tissues in small numbers; if necessary they develop into mononuclear macrophages. Macrophage activity additionally recruits pro-

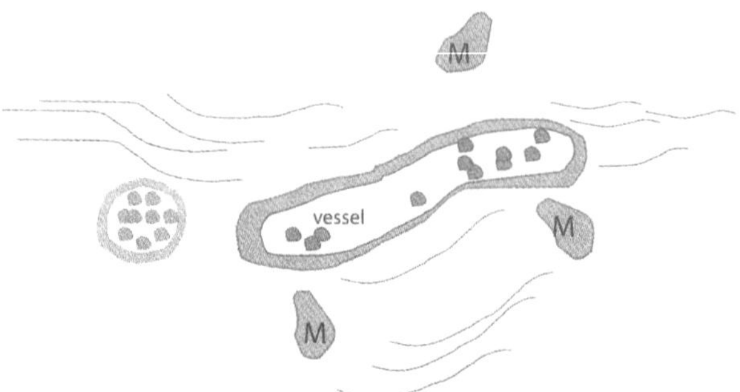

Fig. 2. Pre-existing macrophages (*M*) rest in capsular tissues and become activated for repair mechanisms

genitor cells from the hematopoietic system via the blood stream. Progenitor cells then differentiate into macrophages (Fig. 2). Macrophages may have one or more nuclei; they are cells able to incorporate material and to eliminate it by digestion and/or transportation. Macrophages may fuse with other macrophages and progenitor cells to form multinuclear giant cells; these are able to incorporate particles too big for macrophages. Also, in case of abundant occurrence of particulate foreign material, the tissue contains a high number of giant cells. A group of giant cells often covers particles too large to be incorporated.

The Uptake of Wear Products into the Tissue

The particles liberated from the articulating surfaces are taken up by the joint capsule (Fig. 3). Three layers of tissue forming the rebuilt capsule can be described. A cell-rich, relatively thin layer forms the surface of the capsule; in some areas it resembles the original joint capsule due to the lining of synovial or synovial-like cells. The second layer is characterized by centrifugally orientated bands of fibrous tissue that separate areas of high vascularization. A gradual increase of fibrous tissue leads to the outer layer mainly formed by fibrous tissues.

The development of a periprosthetic foreign body reaction is initiated by the continuous production of particles. In the early stages after introduction of an implant, the number of accumulated particles seems to be rather moderate. The following granulomatous reaction seems not to significantly influence the regular production of the lubricating synovia [77].

With time we observe a thickening of the capsular tissue. The abrasion of wear particles due to the motion under load reaches a constant level [78] which may increase with the occurrence of third-bodies (bone fragments, bone cement, contrast media, metal wear, corrosion products), hard enough to roughen the articulating surfaces. This permanent replenishment of particles demands a continuous supply of phagocytes which accumulate to granu-

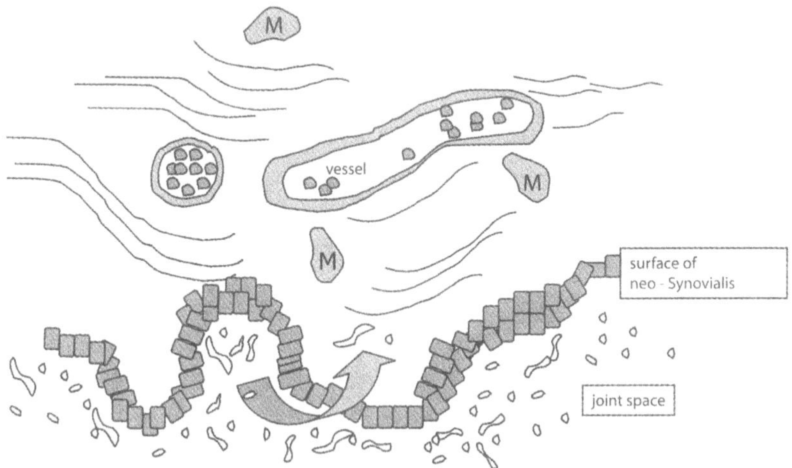

Fig. 3. Wear particles from the joint fluid are taken up by the neo-synovialis

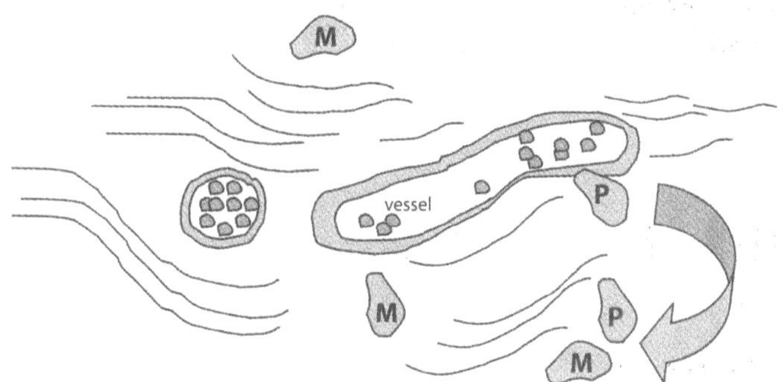

Fig. 4. Further progenitor cells (*P*) enter the capsule from the bloodstream and become macrophages (*M*)

lomas (Figs. 4, 5). Thus the growth of the foreign body granulomas is inevitably fuelled by the regular use of the joint. The growing granulomata undergo fibrosis and the tissue of the capsule becomes more rigid and narrows the joint space.

Growth of granulomas and scarring result in necrosis, especially in the center of the granulomas. Often, necroses of the joint capsule break open, and paste-like detritus empties into the joint space. This leads to further irritation and impairment of function of the inner synovial layers of the capsule. Obviously, necrotic masses are an additional stimulus for granuloma formation.

Mechanical instability of the anchoring parts of the devices adds fragments and abrasion products of bone cement as well as bone debris to the foreign body reaction. Fluid in the joint and in the connected gaps between the implant parts and bone is pumped to and fro and thereby mixed. In the

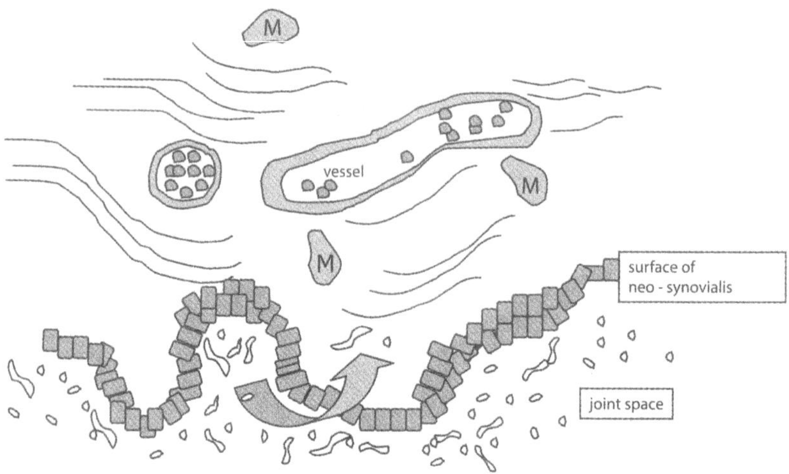

Fig. 5. Excessive wear released into the joint space is taken up by neo-synovial cells lining the capsular surface. Thus, the particles enter the tissues and cause recruitment of further macrophages

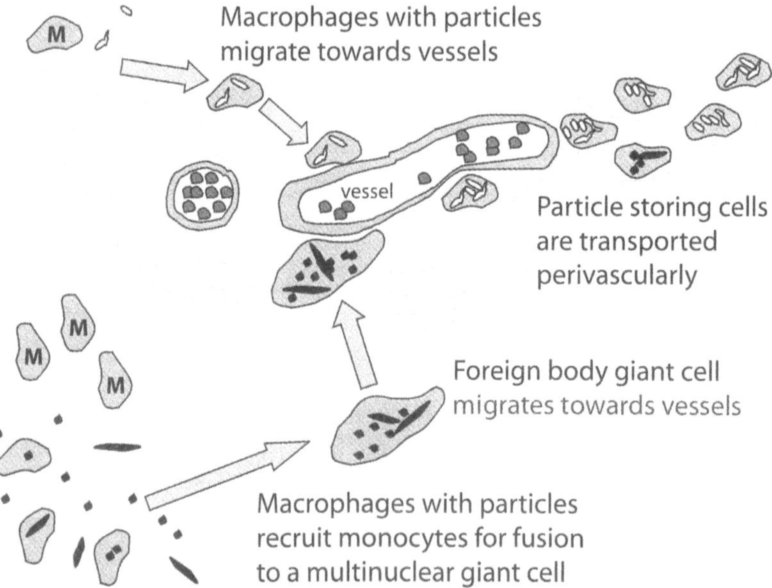

Fig. 6. Macrophages and foreign-body cells loaden with particles migrate towards a vessel. Particles are frequently found within the peri-vascular lymph spaces. The particles are transported within the lymphatic system and become transported to distant sites

process of loosening, bone resorption is induced by the spread of the granulation tissue (see below).

Macrophages and/or giant cells with phagocytosed particles migrate towards the perivascular lymph spaces (Fig. 6). The accumulations along these routes as well as the observed storage of particles in lymph nodes are to be understood as a transport mechanism intended to eliminate the foreign material. Obviously, this mechanism is limited to a certain number of particles that is unknown to us. We know, however, that at a certain time prior to aseptic loosening this cleaning mechanism can decompensate.

Metal wear particles are usually stored in mononuclear macrophages, seldom in foreign body giant cells. The macrophages accumulate perivascularly or form stretched islands in fibrous tissues; massive numbers of particles lead to voluminous granulomas of macrophages that may become necrotic.

The kind of phagocytes storing UHMWPE wear particles is directly connected to the wide range of particle size. On the one hand, there are hip joints that apparently release particles only in the size of one micron and smaller (submicron wear). On the other hand, we also find heavy wearing joints with a high rate of abrasive and adhesive wear as well as sub-surface delaminations (1 mm^2-large scales). It is obvious that according to different sizes the cellular reaction is different. Macrophages incorporate particles of dimensions up to about 5 µm. Foreign body giant cells incorporate all sizes of particles up to about 50 µm. Big flakes and fragments become engulfed by several giant cells. UHMWPE-wear storing cells accumulate in granulomas that may reach volumes of some 5–10 cm^3.

PMMA-wear particles also cover a wide range of sizes and, similar to UHMWPE, this material is stored in macrophages and giant cells. The fragments found in the interfaces of the implant anchorage often are bigger than polyethylene wear. Fragments of PMMA-pearls and parts of the polymerized matrix can clearly be differentiated. Particle storing macrophages accumulate in islands within fibrous tissue, perivascular transport is often observed. Their solubility in, e.g., xylene, makes PMMA particles impossible to detect in regular paraffin sections. Often the swollen, foamy appearance of the cytoplasm of macrophages and some grayish coloring are the only hints that macrophages might be filled with fine PMMA debris. In frozen sections, however, fat stains can be applied, and the incorporated PMMA debris then becomes visible as an almost homogeneous mass within the macrophages.

Contrast media as part of the bone cement become liberated after destruction of the PMMA matrix due to fragmentation of the cement. The main source is abrasion of the cement pieces against each other or against the neighboring bone and the implant. As a secondary product of PMMA abrasion, they are additionally involved in the reactions to other materials, e.g., PMMA, PE, or metal. They are stored in macrophages and giant cells, often together with other material and are transported perivascularly.

Ti-alloy corrosion products are mechanically liberated from the metal/ bone interfaces either as larger plates or fragmented into smaller pieces. Thus they are to be found in macrophages as well as in giant cells. The tissue reactions observed seemed to be more influenced by the acidity of the corrosion process than by these particles [63].

The Spread of Particles

All tissues surrounding the implant are clearly connected by some sort of communication system through which, for example, cells and other substances, such as bacteria but obviously also particles of the implant materials, can find their way from one region to another. The products of material disintegration and wear become distributed with time around the whole area of the endoprosthesis, regardless of the site they were produced at. That means that the joint space, tissue of the joint capsule, the implant/bone interface and the bone marrow must be connected by a communication system in which the particles can spread [62].

If the particles are generated in the joint or at the head-taper interface, they will be primarily phagocytosed by the joint capsule from which further spread proceeds to the implant/bone interface and the bone marrow. If the particles originate from the anchoring surfaces or "debonded" implant components, they will primarily come into contact with the tissue at the implant/bone interface and spread from there to the bone marrow, the joint space, and to further remote implant/bone interfaces [64, 71].

At the time of revision surgery, the process of wear and loosening has often advanced to such an extent that wear products of all materials can be found in the granulomas. At that stage it is almost impossible to determine the material or location responsible for the onset of granuloma formation [62].

Several mechanisms are believed to be responsible for the distribution of wear particles to regions remote from their origin:
1. Transport via the perivascular lymph spaces
   Monocytes may enter tissues and macrophages are known to eliminate nondigestible materials. They migrate towards vessels and transport the material via perivascular lymphatics to regional lymph nodes (Fig. 6). If these barriers are overpassed, a further systemic distribution to organs of the reticulo-endothelial system has been described [5, 10, 12, 22, 24, 29, 40, 48, 49, 50, 58, 75, 76].
2. Continuous perifocal invasion into the vicinity
   The invasion of proliferating tissues and simultaneous replacement of pre-existent structures is well known in tumor formation (growth "per continuitatem") and in rheumatoid arthritis ("aggressive granulomas"). This mechanism also becomes active with foreign body granulomas, which expand into the surroundings. The macrophages transport the incorporated wear products centrifugally to fibrous tissues, muscles, and bone marrow.
3. Passive dissemination via open communicating spaces
   Particles become mixed with the body fluids (e.g., joint lubricant) and are distributed to areas distant from their point of origin [62]. Mechanically produced gaps allow spread of fluid from the joint cavity to distant interfaces. Communicating spaces have also been termed "effective joint space" [44].

In a long-lasting artificial joint replacement, a slow but continuous growth of the joint capsule appears to be tolerated. Here, foreign body granulomas do not interfere with the interfaces between implant devices and bone nor the bone marrow; thus the load transfer from the implants to the bone structures established during the phase of stabilization is maintained [60, 65, 79]. Perivascular transportation and storage balance the production of wear debris. However, in most joint replacements this delicate equilibrium may decompensate after a nonpredictable time of function. The development of granulomatous reactions to particulate wear debris in the direct vicinity of bone will inevitably induce bone resorption. As already described, the granulomatous reactions may develop primarily at or may spread secondarily to the implant interface; granulomas also may first develop in the marrow spaces of spongious bone without connection to the implant/bone interface, but extend later there and induce osteolysis. As we always find granulomatous tissue with abundant particle-laden macrophages and giant cells in the osteolytic defects, it seems obvious that the phagocytic reaction is responsible for the formation of osteolyses. It seems quite unlikely that osteolyses in the surrounding area of mechanically stable joint implants can be produced in the absence of wear particles. Load to stable anchored devices does not produce pressure gradients able to destabilize the implant/bone interface. The incidence of osteolytic defects would be enormously high if variations in pressure would be as effective as hypothesized [2, 3, 44, 55–57, 80–82]. It is, however, possible that changes in volume and pressure due to implant loosening support the development of granuloma-induced osteolyses.

Foreign Body Granulomata Induce Bone Resorption

Histochemical analysis of cells in tissue cultures as well as of tissue sections has contributed detailed information to the understanding and interpretation of the relationship between wear and osteolysis. Exchange of information between cells is established by chemical substances (synonymously called mediators or cytokines) which cause several different reactions depending on the type of cell and the concurrent existence of other substances (Fig. 7). These mediators have been defined "as soluble products released from one cell that can modulate the activity of other cells" and have "an important role ... in regulating bone remodelling in the adult organism" [4, 9, 18, 84]. Their synergistic nature and efficacy has been described [51, 53].

Macrophages and osteoblasts, and perhaps also fibroblasts, are activated by foreign-body particles to produce mediators that stimulate bone resorption and reduce bone formation [23, 32, 38, 59]. In areas of remodelling there are always active osteoblasts and osteoclasts to be seen.

It is generally accepted that the lining cells which cover the bone surface are resting osteoblasts [4, 17, 30, 31, 42, 43, 84] (Fig. 8). They control the turnover of bone in regular bone remodelling and may be activated by strain, injury, or mediators released from cells, for instance from other osteoblasts.

In the tissues directly adjacent to the bone (hematopoietic and fat marrow), a certain number of osteoclast-progenitor cells are present that originate as mononuclear mesenchymal stem cells from the bone marrow and

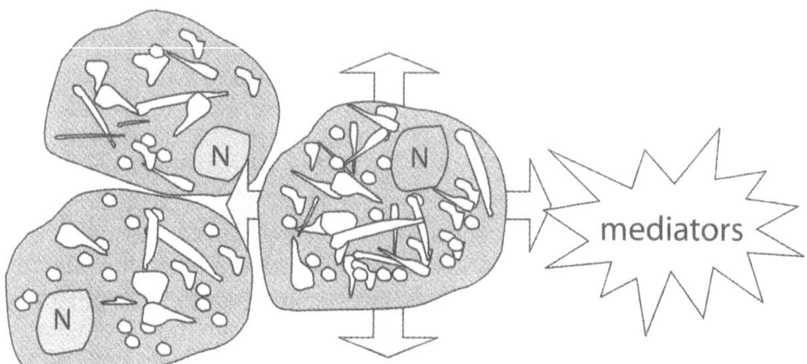

Fig. 7. The frustrated attempts of macrophages to digest particulate foreign material results in the liberation of lysosomal enzymes and mediators. Further on cells undergo apoptosis and necrotic material as well as particles cause recruitment of new macrophages

Macrophages and foreign body giant cells reach the bone marrow

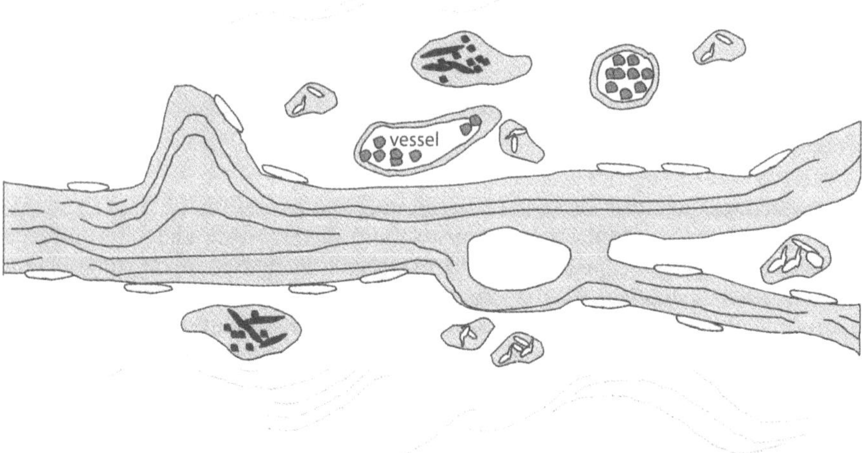

Fig. 8. Macrophages and foreign body cells come into contact with bone marrow and bone. This is due to transportation as well as to production of debris in the bone-implant interface

from the blood. Recruited and activated by osteoblast-derived mediators, pre-osteoclasts are stimulated to join to colonies and fuse into multinucleated osteoclasts. These become powerful cells by accumulation of activity of 10 up to 100 osteoclast precursors (represented by their nuclei) [42]. For a long time it has been stated that progenitor cells (of osteoblasts or osteoclasts) are highly differentiated and have no ability to reproduce themselves. Osteoclast progenitors are not yet capable of resorbing bone [17]. Osteoblasts were shown to mediate the interleukin-1 stimulation of osteoclast activity [53].

Osteoblasts are thought to attract osteoclasts to start their activity at certain points of the bone surface; however, the mechanisms of where to start and of the extent of resorption are not yet completely understood. One explanation is the production of collagenase by some neighboring osteoblasts to dissolve the nonmineralized collagen surface membrane of bone, thus exposing an area of mineralized bone for osteoclast attack [4, 84]. Osteoclasts settle on the de-collagenized surfaces and resorb bone mineral and matrix.

The resorbing activity of osteoclasts liberates constituents of the dissolved bone matrix which now enhance osteoblast activity. Consequently, osteoblasts cover empty lacunae and surfaces and produce osteoid on the surfaces presumably according to a certain need directed by a pattern of strain. Mineralization of the osteoid restores a functional stability of the new structures.

Through this mutual stimulation, bone resorption as well as new bone formation are active at the same time. This allows the bone mass to be maintained. The exchange of stimuli has been termed "coupling mechanism." The places of the two counteracting activities may either be in close vicinity (for instance in a Howship's lacuna) or on opposing bone surfaces (for instance of a trabeculum). Depending on the mode of stimulation, the bone forming and the bone resorbing activities balance each other or one of the two coupled but counteracting effects dominate: Physiologic bone remodelling keeps the balance while new bone formation predominates in fracture healing and "secondary fixation" of endoprostheses; but bone resorption prevails in osteoporosis, bone atrophy, and osteolytic lesions.

In fracture healing and osseointegration of implants the increased bone turnover ends or at least retards significantly with the restoration of the bone structures to "sufficient," if not complete, function [66]. Ziegler [84] assumes that dose-dependent effects of local mediator concentrations and/or the regulation of extracellular calcium concentrations, after, for instance, healing of a fracture and restoration or adaptation to the change of load transfer, will act on the termination or retardation of the local remodelling process.

Progenitor cells for macrophages are also of hematopoietic origin. They migrate into the vicinity of bone where the progenitor cell becomes a pluripotent macrophage, which further differentiates either into a "resident" macrophage (histiocyte, type A cell of the synovium) or into an inflammatory, "exudate" macrophage. The latter may form multinucleated giant cells [42]. The important functional characteristic of the macrophage is the ingestion of particulate material in order to eliminate the material by digestion. The macrophage carries several degrading chemicals for digestion (lysosomal enzymes) and is able to maintain an increased production thereof.

The recruitment of macrophages and the formation of multinucleated giant cells is comparable to osteoclast formation because here stimuli for accumulation and fusion are necessary too. These stimuli come from infection, tissue injury, foreign materials, necroses, and immune reactions. Papadimitriou [36] showed in animal experiments that "fusion is much more frequent between macrophages with exudate characteristics." It has been shown by Bennett [6] that in in vitro experiments frustrated ingestion by "resident" macrophages stimulates their proliferation.

The tissue macrophage has a remarkable life span of months or years [4], while the half-life of murine foreign body multinucleated giant cells was reported to be only a few days [37].

Intensive research has been undertaken to understand the pathology of basic inflammatory processes such as foreign body reactions to wear particles or corrosion products and immunologic reactions to metals or polymers. In foreign-body-induced as well as immunologic reactions, macrophages secrete a large number of biologically active substances [18–21, 31, 32, 46, 83]. These either act directly on the foreign materials or are mediators to be distributed in the tissue and to stimulate other effects. Additionally, macrophages realize large particles as too big for incorporation and attempt to dissolute their surfaces. They are able to maintain a long-lasting contact with biocompatible surfaces by excretion of extracellular protein matrix. On the other hand, failed attempts of incorporation or contact (probably of less biocompatible materials) most probably lead to the formation of multinucleated giant cells. In this process, additional macrophages become attracted by excretion of mediators; they are stimulated to accumulate and to merge into multinucleated giant cells [83, 84]. Interesting to note is the report of Papadimitriou et al. [37] that macrophages which had ingested a substance from a plastic surface became unable to fuse; however, the macrophages (progenitor cells) formed high numbers of multinucleated giant cells. Multinucleated giant cells are reported not to lose the ability of the original macrophages to secrete lysosomal enzymes. This parallels the secretory activity of osteoclasts.

As concluded by Rae [42] and Athanasou [4], macrophages and multinucleated giant cells excrete agents that on the one hand have potential to dissolve bone mineral and matrix, and on the other hand obviously stimulate osteoclast formation.

The macrophage or the multinucleated giant cell, however, if compared to the osteoclast, lacks the typical morphologic characteristics of a ruffled membrane and appears– in in vitro experiments – to be less effective in bone resorption. Macrophages are reported not to be able to produce Howship's lacunae but to attack areas of the bone surface only superficially [41]. Whether macrophages are able to resorb bone directly, as stated by several investigators [35, 39, 41], or to even form "resorption bays" [52] or only contribute stimulating mediators, as we would interpret their results, is still a matter of debate. Kadoya and coworkers stated that in culture studies there is uncertainty in differentiating osteoclast-like cells from foreign body giant cells [26]. Further findings that "particle-storing monocytes" are capable of direct bone resorption [27, 28, 38] do not correspond with our histology. We normally observe a very thin layer of (lining-) cells and fibers interposed between the bone-forming or resorbing cells and the particle-laden macrophages of the foreign body granuloma. At least in the light microscopic range, we never saw particle-containing macrophages or foreign-body giant cells directly involved in resorbing or forming bony substance. Direct contact between macrophages and bone, with or without interposition of lining cells alone [27, 28], however, does not warrant the assumption that macrophages are able to directly resorb bone. Obviously the circumstances in in vitro experiments do not exactly imitate in vivo conditions, and conclusions on the basis of theses experiments, therefore, appear to be misleading.

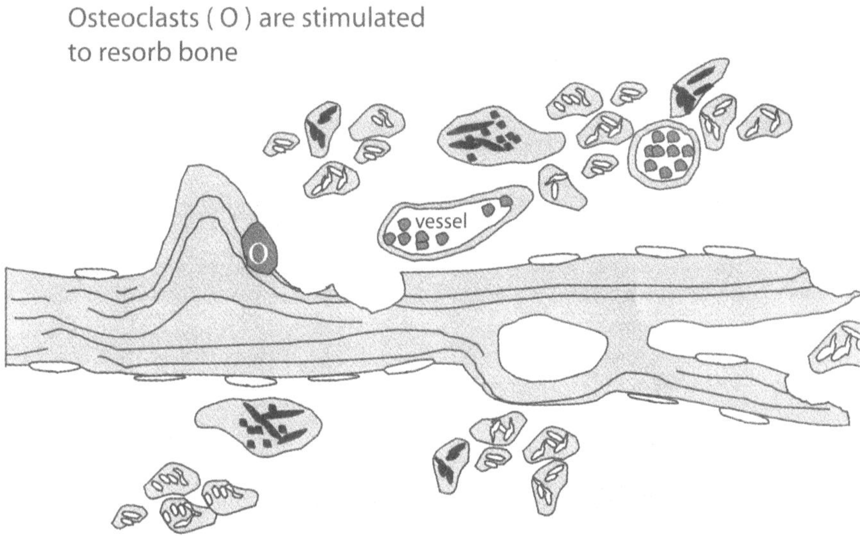

Fig. 9. The release of mediators not only stimulates the formation of foreign body giant cells but also the fusion of precursor cells to osteoclasts. These settle on the surface of bone and resorb the matrix

In total joint replacements, the invasion of a granulation tissue into the implant–bone interface causes changes in the regular remodelling of the implant-carrying bone (Fig. 8). As a response to the foreign material incorporated in macrophages, mediators are released into the surroundings in order to recruit pre-macrophages from the hematopoietic system. However, these mediators obviously also activate the osteoblast–osteoclast activity. An irregularly high number of mononuclear precursor cells reach the borderline between the foreign body granulation tissue, the bone, and the bone marrow. The predominance of osteoclasts over the regular number in bone remodelling overwhelms the repair mechanism. Thus bone is lost in favor of the spread of the granulation tissue and the anchorage of the implant is weakened (Fig. 9).

With the permanent burden of nondigestible wear products, a permanent liberation of mediators by the macrophages maintains osteoclast activity; this process cannot end in the sense of bone healing. In case of cell death, new macrophages become recruited and continue the frustrated digestion and release of mediators. Granuloma formation and subsequent bone loss ultimately result in mechanical instability.

The loss of stability increases the motions of implant and bone surfaces relative to each other. The anchoring implant surfaces become subjected to abrasion and produce wear products directly in the region of implant fixation. At this stage the fixation of the device is definitively lost.

Conclusions

It appears that the recruitment of macrophages in particle-induced granulomatous tissue follows the same pattern as the generation of pre-osteoclasts in fracture healing and remodelling of bone. In fracture healing, Frost [17] supposed that the granulation tissue represents one of the mechanisms releasing mediators that lead to new tissue formation (cartilage and woven bone) by appearance of chondroblasts and osteoblasts.

Incorporation and attempts to digest foreign material may be compared to organization of tissue necrosis and blood clots. The major difference in both events, however, appears to be the insolubility of the foreign material and in consequence the persisting frustration of the macrophages with high production and excretion of lysosomal enzymes and mediators. This may be regarded as the main cause for the imbalance between bone resorption and new formation in favor of osteoclastic resorption. Pazzaglia et al. [39] stated that on the cellular level the main damage is effected by very small metal particles irrespective of their chemical composition, and that particle size and release rate are the most critical factors in the foreign-body reaction.

From this we conclude that the foreign-body-induced granulomas and osteolyses are not self-permeating processes but are fuelled by wear particles. Considering the coupling mechanism, as described above, the wear-particle-induced osteolyses show that osteoclast-activating mediators released by macrophages and foreign-body multinucleated giant cells overrule those mediators stimulating new bone formation. Consequently, an increase of particle concentration as a consequence of particle transport will accelerate bone resorption.

In the first place it is the excessive amount of particles which causes the adverse effects upon bone and other tissues surrounding an artificial joint. Regarding the part in implant loosening, the biochemical nature of the abraded particles seems to be of minor importance. Also the shape of the wear products appears to be a secondary factor. Ideally, neither articulation, modularity of devices, nor implant anchorage should be the source of wear. But the articulation will always produce wear on physical principles. One should therefore take advantage of all possibilities to reduce the production of wear particles in the joint bearing as well as at the anchoring surfaces.

As particles are transported via the parenchymatic system to all places in the body, the systemic effects will probably gain more significance with increasing use.

References

1. Anthony PP, Gie GA, Howie CR, Ling RSM (1990) Localised endosteal bone lysis in relation to the femoral components of cemented total hip arthroplasties. J Bone Joint Surg 72-B:971–979
2. Aspenberg P, Van der Vis HM (1998) Fluid pressure may cause periprosthetic osteolysis – particles are not the only thing. Acta Orthop Scand 69:1–4
3. Aspenberg P, Van Der Vis HM (1998) Migration, particles, and fluid pressure: a discussion of causes of prosthetic loosening. Clin Orthop 352:75–80

4. Athanasou NA (1996) Current concepts review: cellular biology of bone-resorbing cells. J Bone Jount Surg [Am] 87-A:1097–112
5. Baslé MF, Bertrand G, Guyetant S, Chappard D, Lesourd M (1996) Migration of metal and polyethylene particles from articular prostheses may generate lymphadenopathy with histiocytes. J Biomed Mater Res 30:157–64
6. Bennett S, Por, SB, Cooley MA, Breit SN (1993) In vitro replication dynamics of human culture-derived macrophages in a long-term serum-free system. J Immunol 150:2364–2371
7. Bermann G (1997) In vivo Messung der Belastung von Hüftimplantaten. Verlag Dr. Köster, Berlin
8. Bloebaum RD, Beeks D, Dorr LD, Savory CG, DuPont JA, Hofmann AA (1994) Complications with hydroxyapatite particulate separation in total hip arhroplasty. Clin Orthop Rel Res 298:19–26
9. Bonewald LF, Mundy MD (1990) Role of transforming growth factor beta in bone remodeling. Clin Orthop Rel Res 250:261–276
10. Bos I, Johannisson R, Lohrs U, Lindner B, Seydel U (1990) Comparative investigations of regional lymph and pseudocapsules after implantation of joint endoprostheses. Pathol Res Pract 186:707–16
11. Campbell P, Schmalzried T, Amstutz HC (1992) Special staining supports the presence of submicron UHMWPE wear debris in periprosthetic tissues. Implant Retrieval Symposium, Society for Biomaterials – Transactions, Society for Biomaterials, Minneapolis, pp 31
12. Case CP, Langkamer VG, James C Palmer MR, Kemp AJ, Heap PF, Solomon L (1994) Widespread dissemination of metal debris from implants, J Bone Joint Surg 76-B:701–712
13. Charnley J (1970) Acrylic cement in orthopaedic surgery. Livingstone, Edinburgh – London
14. Collier JP, Surprenant VA, Jensen RE, Mayor MB (1991) Corrosion at the interface of cobalt-alloy heads on titanium-alloy stems. Clin Orthop 271:305–312
15. Collier JP, Surprenant VA, Jensen RE, Mayor MB, Surprenant HP (1992) Corrosion between the components of modular femoral hip prostheses. J Bone Joint Surg 74-B:511–517
16. Davidson JA, Poggie RA, Mishra AK (1994) Abrasive wear of ceramic, metal, and UHMWPE bearing surfaces from third-body bone, PMMA bone cement, and titanium debris. Biomed Mater Eng 4:213–229
17. Frost HM (1989) The biology of fracture healing – an overview for clinicians, part 1. Clin Orthop Rel Res 248:283–293
18. Goldring MB, Goldring SR (1990) Skeletal tissue response to cytokines. Clin Orthop Rel Res 258:245–278
19. Goldring SR, Jasty M, Roelke MS, Rourke CM, Bringhurst FR, Harris WH (1986) Formation of a synovial-like membrane at the bone-cement interface. Arthritis and Rheumatism 29:836–842
20. Goldring SR, Schiller AL, Roelke M, Rourke CM, O'Neill DA, Harris WH (1983) The synovial-like membrane at the bone-cement interface in loose total hip replacements and its proposed role in bone lysis. J Bone Joint Surg 65-A:575–584
21. Goodman SB (1994) The effects of micromotion and particulate materials on tissue differentiation. Acta Orthop Scand 65, Suppl 258:1–43
22. Heilmann K, Diezel PB, Rossner JA, Brinkmann KA (1975) Morphological studies in tissues surrounding alloarthroplastic joints. Virchows Arch A Path Anat Histol 366:93–106
23. Herman JH, Sowder WG, Anderson D, Appel AM, Hopson CN (1989) Polymethylmethacrylate-induced release of bone-resorbing factors. J Bone Joint Surg 71-A:1530–1541
24. Hicks DG, Judkins AR, Sickel JZ et al (1996) Granularhistiocytosis of pelvic lymph nodes following total hip arthroplasty: the presence of wear debris, cytokine production, and immunologically activated macrophages. J Bone Joint Surg [Am] 78-A:482–96
25. Jones SMG, Pinder IM, Morran CG, Malcolm AJ (1992) Polyethylene wear in uncemented knee replacements. J Bone Joint Surg 74-Br:18–22
26. Kadoya Y, Al-Saffar N, Kobayashi A, Revell PA (1994) The expression of osteoclast markers on foreign body giant cells. Bone Mineral 27:85–96
27. Kadoya Y, Kobayashi A, Ohashi H (1998) Wear and osteolysis in total joint replacenents. Acta Orthop Scand Suppl. No. 278 69:1–16

28. Kadoya Y, Revell PA, Al-Saffar N, Kobayashi A, Scott G, Freemann MAR (1996) Bone formation and bone resorption in failed total joint arthroplasties: histomorphometric analysis with histochemical and immunohistochemical technique. J Orthop Research 14:473–482
29. Langkamer VG, Case CP, Heap P, Taylor, Collins C, Pearse M, Solomon L (1992) Systemic distribution of wear debris after hip replacement – a cause for concern? J Bone Joint Surg 74-B:831–839
30. Lind M (1998) Growth factor stimulation of bone healing – effects on osteoblasts, osteotomies and implant fixation. Thesis. Acta Orthop Scand Suppl 283(69)
31. Lind M, Trindade MCD, Yaszay B, Goodman SB, Smith RL (1998) Effects of particulate debris on macrophage-dependent fibroblast stimulation in coculture. J Bone Joint Surg 80-B:924–930
32. Maloney WJ, James RE, Smith RL (1996) Human macrophage response to retrieved titanium alloy particles in vitro. Clin Orthop Rel Res 322:268–278
33. Manley MT, Serekian P (1994) Wear debris. An environmental issue in total joint replacement. Clin Orthop Rel Res 298:137–146
34. Morscher EW, Hefti A, Aebi U (1998) Severe osteolysis after third body wear due to hydroxyapatite particles from acetabular cup coating. J Bone Joint Surg 80-B:267–272
35. Mundy GR, Altman AJ, Gondek MD, Bandelin JG (1977) Direct resorption of bone by human monocytes. Science 196:1109–1111
36. Papadimitriou JM (1979) The role of resident and exudate macrophages in multinucleate giant cell formation. J Pathol 128:93–97
37. Papadimitriou JM, Sforsina D, Papaelias L (1973) Kinetics of multinucleate giant cell formation and their modification by various agents in foreign body reactions. Am J Pathol 73:349–64
38. Pazzaglia UE, Ceciliani L, Wilkinson MJ, Dell'Orbo C (1985) Involvement of metal particles in loosening of metal-plastic prostheses. Arch Orthop Trauma Surg 104:164–174
39. Pazzaglia UE, Dell'Orbo C, Wilkinson MJ (1987) The foreign body reaction in total hip arthroplasties – a correlated light-microscopy, SEM, and TEM study. Arch Orthop Trauma Surg 106:209–219
40. Peoc'h M, Pasquier D, Ducros V, Moulin C, Bost F, Faure C, Pasquier B (1996) Systemic granulomatous reaction in hip prosthesis. Apropos two anatomical cases. Rev Chir Orthop Reparatrice Appar Mot 82:564–567
41. Quinn J, Joyner C, Triffitt JT, Athanasou NA (1992) Polymethylmethacrylate – induced inflammatory macrophages resorb bone. J Bone Joint Surg 74-B:652–658
42. Rae T (1986) The macrophage response to implant materials – with special reference to those used in orthopedics. In: Williams DF (ed) Critical reviews in biocompatibility. CRC Press, Boca Raton, pp 97–126
43. Resch H, Battmann A (1995) Die Bedeutung von Wachstumsfaktoren und Zytokinen im Knochenstoffwechsel und Remodeling. Osteologie 4:137–144
44. Schmalzried TP, Jasty M, Harris WH (1992) Periprosthetic bone loss in total hip arthroplasty – polyethylene wear debris and the concept of the effective joint space. J Bone Joint Surg 74-A:849–863
45. Schmalzried TP, Kwong LM, Jasty M, Sedlacek RC, Haire TC, O'Connor DO, Bragdon CR, Kabo JM, Malcolm AJ, Harris WH (1992) The mechanism of loosening of cemented acetabular components in total hip arthroplasty. Analysis of specimens retrieved at autopsy. Clin Orthop 274:60–78
46. Sedel L, Simeon J, Meunier A, Vilette, Launay SM (1992) Prostaglandin E2 level in tissue surrounding aseptic failed total hips. Effects of materials. Arch Orthop Trauma Surg 111:255–258
47. Semlitsch M, Willert HG (1995) Implant materials for hip endoprostheses: old proofs and new trends. Arch Orthop Trauma Surg 114:61–67
48. Shea KG, Bloebaum RD, Avent JM, Birk GT, Samuelson KM (1996) Analysis of lymph nodes for polyethylene particles in patients who have had a primary joint replacement. J Bone Joint Surg [Am] 78-A:497–504
49. Shea KG, Lundeen GA, Bloebaum RD, Bachus KN, Zou L (1997) Lymphoreticular dissemination of metal particles after primary joint replacements. Clin Orthop Rel Res 338:219–226
50. Shinto Y, Uchida A, Yoshikawa H et al (1993) Inguinal lymphadenopathy due to metal release from a prosthesis: a case report. J Bone Joint Surg [Br] 75-B:266–269
51. Stashenko P, Dewhirst FD, Peros WJ, Kent RL, Ago JM (1987) Synergistic interactions between interleukin-1, tumor necrosis factor, and lymphotoxin in bone resorption. J Immunol 138:1464–1468

52. Teitelbaum SL, Stewart CC, Kahn AJ (1979) Rodent peritoneal macrophages as bone resorbing cells. Calcif Tiss Int 27:255–261
53. Thompson BM, Saklatvala J, Chambers TJ (1986) Osteoblasts mediate interleukin-1 stimulation of bone resorption by rat osteoclasts. J Exper Med 164:104–112
54. Thomson BM, Mundy GR, Chambers TJ (1987) Tumor necrosis factor a and β induce osteoblastic cells to stimulate osteoclastic bone resorption. J Immunol 138:775–779
55. Van der Vis HM, Aspenberg P, de Kleine R, Tigchelaar W, van Noorden CJF (1998) Short periods of oscillating fluid pressure directed at a titanium-bone interface in rabbits lead to bone lysis. Acta Orthop Scand 69:5–10
56. Van der Vis HM, Marti RK, Tigchelaar W, Schüller HM, Van Noorden CJF (1997) Benign cellular responses in rats to differne wear particles in intra-articular and intramedullary environments. J Bone Jouint Surg 79-B:837–843
57. Van Der Vis HM, Aspenberg P, Marti RK, Tigchelaar W, van Noorden CJF (1998) Fluid pressure causes bone resorption in a rabbit model of prosthetic loosening. Clin Orthop Rel Res 350:201–208
58. Vernon-Roberts B, Freeman MAR (1976) In: Schaldach M, Hohmann D (eds) Morphological and analytical studies of the tissues adjacent to joint prostheses: investigations into the causes of loosening of prostheses. In: Engineering in medicine, Vol. 2. Advances in artificial hip and knee joint technology. Springer Verlag, pp 148–186
59. Wang JT, Harada Y, Goldring SR (1993) Biological mechanisms involved in the pathogenesis of aseptic loosening after total joint replacement. Sem Arthroplasty 4:215–222
60. Willert HG (1973) Tissue reactions around joint implants and bone cement. In: Chapchal G (ed) Arthroplasty of the hip. Georg Thieme Verlag, Stuttgart, pp 11–21
61. Willert HG, Bertram H, Buchhorn GH (1990) Osteolysis in alloarthroplasty of the hip – the role of UHMW polyethylene wear. Clin Orthop Rel Res 258:95–107
62. Willert HG, Bertram H, Buchhorn GH (1990) Osteolysis in alloarthroplasty of the hip – the role of bone cement fragmentation. Clin Orthop Rel Res 258:108–121
63. Willert HG, Brobäck LG, Buchhorn GH, Jensen PH, Köster G, Lang I, Ochsner P, Schenk R (1996) Crevice corrosion of cemented titanium-alloy stems in total hip replacements. Clin Orthop Rel Res 333:51–75
64. Willert HG, Buchhorn GH (1993) Particle disease due to wear of ultrahigh molecular weight polyethylene – findings from retrieval studies. In: Morrey B (ed) Biological, material, and mechanical considerations of joint replacement; current concepts and future direction. Raven Press, New York, pp 87–102
65. Willert HG, Buchhorn GH (1994) Overview of long-term interface response. In: NIH Consensus Development Conference on Total Hip Replacement. National Institutes of Health, Bethesda, Maryland USA, pp 71–82
66. Willert HG, Buchhorn GH (1999) Osseointegration of cemented and noncemented implants in artificial hip replacement. Long-term findings in man. J Long-Term Effects Medical Implants 9:113–130
67. Willert HG, Buchhorn GH (2000) Cement bone interface: Histological analysis of the interface. In: Learmonth ID (ed) Interfaces in total hip arthroplasty. Springer, London, pp 33–43
68. Willert HG, Buchhorn GH, Göbel D, Köster G, Schaffner S, Schenk R, Semlitsch M (1996) Wear behaviour and histopathology of classic cemented metal on metal hip endoprostheses. Clin Orthop Rel Res 329S:160–186
69. Willert HG, Buchhorn GH, Hess T (1989) Die Bedeutung von Abrieb und Materialermüdung bei der Prothesenlockerung an der Hüfte. Orthopäde 18:350–369
70. Willert HG, Buchhorn GH, Semlitsch M (1981) Recognition and identification of wear products in the surrounding tissues of artificial joint prostheses. In: Dumbleton JJ (ed) Tribology of natural and artificial joints. Elsevier Sci Publ Comp, Amsterdam, pp 381–419
71. Willert HG, Buchhorn GH, Semlitsch M (1993) Particle disease due to wear of metal alloys – findings from retrieval studies. In: Morrey B (ed) Biological, material, and mechanical considerations of joint replacement; current concepts and future direction. Raven Press, New York, pp 129–146
72. Willert HG, Lintner F (1987) Morphologie des Implantatlagers bei zementierten und nichtzementierten Gelenkimplantaten. Langenbecks Arch Chir 372:447–455
73. Willert HG, Müller K, Semlitsch M (1979) The morphology of polymethylmethacrylate (PMMA) bone cement surface structures and causes of their origin. Arch Orthop Traumat Surg 94:265–292
74. Willert HG, Puls P (1972) Die Reaktion des Knochens auf Knochenzement bei der Allo-Arthroplastik der Hüfte. Arch orthop und Unfall-Chir 72:33–71

75. Willert HG, Semlitsch M (1972) Histopathology associated with polymers and metals in total hip replacements. Gordon Conference on Science and Technology of Biomaterials. Tilton/USA 14–18.08 (reprint Sulzer Brothers Limited, Winterthur)
76. Willert HG, Semlitsch M (1976) Reactions of the articular capsule to artificial joint prostheses. In: Williams D (ed) Biocompatibility of implant materials. Sector, London, pp 40–48
77. Willert HG, Semlitsch M (1977) Reactions of the articular capsule to wear products of artificial joint prostheses. J Biomed Mat Res 11:157–164
78. Willert HG, Semlitsch M, Buchhorn GH, Kriete U (1978) Materialverschleiß und Gewebereaktion bei künstlichen Gelenken. Orthopäde 7:62–83
79. Willert HG, Puls P (1972) Die Reaktion des Knochens auf Knochenzement bei der Allo-Arthroplastik der Hüfte. Arch orthop und Unfall-Chir 72:33–71
80. Wroblewski BM (1994) Osteolysis due to particle wear debris following total arthroplasty: the role of high-density polyethylene. Instr Course Lect 43:289–94
81. Wroblewski BM (1994) Osteolysis due to particle wear debris following total hip arthroplasty: the role of high-density polyethylene. Instr Course Lect 43:289–294
82. Wroblewski BM (1997) Wear of high-density polyethylene socket in total hip arthroplasty and its role in endosteal cavitation. Proc Inst Mech Eng 211:109–118
83. Xu JW, Konnttinen YT, Lassus J, Natah S, Ceponis, A, Solovieta S, Aspenberg P, Santavirta S (1996) Tumor necrosis factor alpha in loosening of total hip replacements. Clin Exp Rheumatol 14:643–638
84. Ziegler R (1995) Der Knochen und seine Erkrankungen. parts 1–4. Dtsch med Wschr 120:531–532, 571–572, 1091–1092, 1251–1252

Effect of PMMA Creep and Prosthesis Surface Finish on the Behavior of a Tapered Cemented Total Hip Stem

TIMOTHY L. NORMAN

Introduction

The failure or success of a hip prosthesis is dependent on many factors. This manuscript addresses the effect of polymethylmethacrylate (PMMA) creep and prosthesis surface finish on stem motion and fixation and on the stem-cement interface stress state. Our interest in this area derives from a dichotomy that exists in current design philosophies. One philosophy promotes bonding, thereby favoring a rough surface (Harris 1992). Another philosophy promotes debonding by creating a polished surface (Ling 1992). In the Harris philosophy, a matte surface finish is permitted, while a Ling philosophy accepts a polished surface finish. The dichotomy in design philosophies is the polarized opinion between the interface conditions of these two positions. In the Harris philosophy, a debonded stem is unacceptable, and in the Ling philosophy, a debonded stem is acceptable.

Historically, in 1970, Charnley addressed the stem-cement interface conditions when he said that "acrylic cement has no adhesive properties to steel or wet bone" and "there is no adhesion between the polished surface of the prosthesis and the cement." Charnley also addressed the issue of the geometry of the stem when he said, "the tapered stem of the prosthesis is very suitable for weight transmission since it will get tighter under load" and that "there is no need to roughen the surface of the stem in the hope of enhancing the mechanical bond between the metal and the cement." Charnley is referring to what we commonly call "taper lock," a mechanical locking that occurs between the cement mantle and the stem due to radial (normal) stem-cement interface stress.

What do we know about total hip replacement (THR) design and failure today? This was clearly illustrated by an NIH consensus in 1994 (NIH 1995) concerning the failure of total hip replacement, where it was stated that although the state of the art pertaining to THR has changed substantially, "the optimum cement-metal interface has yet to be identified." Clinical results from a worldwide multinational study (Older 1997) revealed that the polished tapered stem has performed very well. The 20-year survivorship analysis of 5089 Charnley total hip replacements showed a 90% survivorship for THR and an 84% survivorship for the femoral component alone. These high percentages warrant identification of design features that make this system successful. Research in our laboratory has been conducted to address some of the key issues of polished, tapered, cemented stems: how does bone cement (and bone) creep in vitro; is creep responsible for stem subsidence observed clinically; what is the integrity of the interface for a rough versus smooth stem; and can creep-induced subsidence lead to stable fixation?

Creep of Bone Cement

It is known from numerous publications that PMMA exhibits a mechanical behavior called creep (Schreyer 1972; Saha and Pal 1984; Chwirut 1984). Creep is the continuous yielding of a material under constant load. Creep changes with load level, temperature, and moisture content. Initially, we expect a high and changing creep rate after a rapid increase in the cement strain due to loading. After some time, the creep rate will become constant. The compressive creep behavior of four different cements, two mixing conditions (hand and vacuum), sorption, injection time, and stress level has been investigated in our laboratory using small cylinders measuring 22 mm in length and 12.5 mm in diameter and tested under compression (Norman et al. 1995, 1997).

Figure 1 shows the compressive creep response of the bone cements tested. A stem-cement interface stress level of about 10 MPa or below corresponds to a well-bonded stem as has been shown in a number of experimental and numerical studies. At this low stress level, creep strain is low (~1%), and there is only a small difference between the four cements tested. At higher stem-cement interface stress levels (above 10 MPa), indicative of debonded stems, the difference between the cements grows. Palacos® has the largest creep of the four cements tested, followed by Zimmer®. Simplex and Osteo-

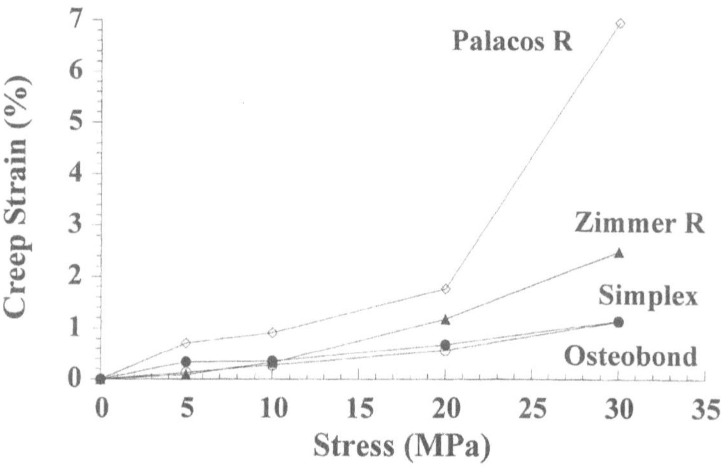

Fig. 1. Creep values of the bone cements tested

bond demonstrate approximately the same amount of creep strain. The compressive creep strain after 24 h ranges from about 1% to about 7%, depending on the cement. Creep tends to be greater in high viscosity cements than low viscosity cements.

The creep behavior of bone cement is an important factor in THR design. Consider a polished stem that debonds because of low stem-cement interface friction. The debonded stem would most likely benefit from a mechanical environment conducive to stem subsidence leading to taper-lock. This scenario is best achieved using a tapered stem with an unsupported distal tip and a cement that has a lower resistance to creep at higher stress levels (e.g., Palacos). If the stem does not debond, then the interface stress and the cement creep remain low. Therefore, the choice of cements for a bonded stem may not matter from a creep point of view.

In Vitro Testing

In vitro tests are conducted to measure stem subsidence, cement mantle strains, and the ability of the stem to achieve taper-lock. The experimental stem was a collarless, polished, tapered stem. The distal tip of each stem was unsupported in all tests to prevent end-bearing conditions that may prevent or slow subsidence. Cement mantle strain was measured using strain gauge carriers manufactured in our lab and attached to the stem. Relative motion between the stem and the bone was measured using a device called DVRT (Differential Variable Reluctance Transducer; Microstrain, Burlington, VT). Palacos® was used in the in vitro tests.

A hip simulator fixture attached to a servo-hydraulic test machine (Materials Testing System, Minneapolis, MN) was designed to simulate single-legged stance (SLS), gait, and stair-climbing in which the load application consisted of femoral head and abductor loading. In addition, a stem pull-out fixture was designed to measure the initial bond strength of the stem in pull-out and the "taper-lock" or "bond" after loading of the reinserted stem.

Results for SLS showed that the displacement of the stem with time (Fig. 2) is indicative of creep-induced subsidence and demonstrates the stick-slip phenomenon, where creep is followed by a reduction in the stem-cement interface normal force, and the stem subsequently slips down into the canal until a force of sufficient magnitude is generated to hold the stem in place. The process is repeated as the stem subsides. The resulting fixation can be measured by a pull-out test. Stem pull-out loads after SLS, cyclic, and stair-climbing loads did not differ significantly from the initial bond strength of the polished stem (Fig. 3). Therefore, the stem taper-lock that exists is just as strong as the original stem-cement bond.

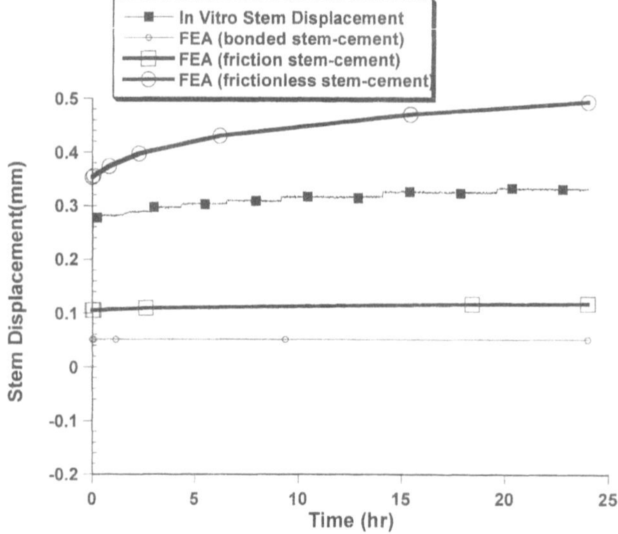

Fig. 2. Experimental and finite element stem displacements with time (From Hustosky et al. 1996)

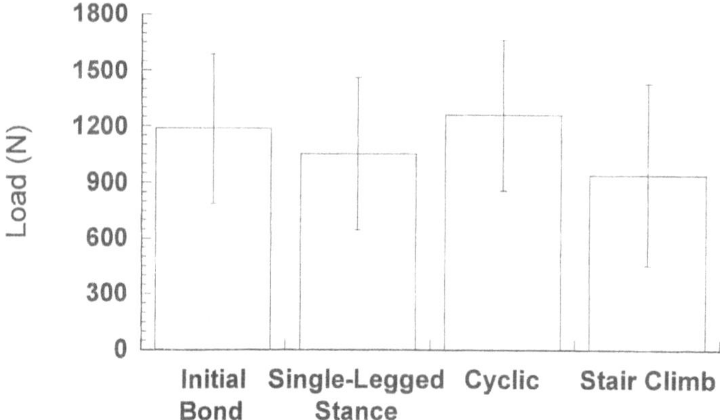

Fig. 3. Stem pull-out loads after initial bonding and after reinsertion and single-legged stance, cyclic and stair-climbing loads. (From Hustosky et al. 1998)

Finite Element Simulations

Using information derived from the experiments, we developed a finite element model that approximated the geometry and simulated the creep response of the bone cement. By comparing in vitro stem displacements and finite element predictions (Fig. 4), it was found that the in vitro matte surface stems exhibit displacements similar to a bonded stem with very little subsi-

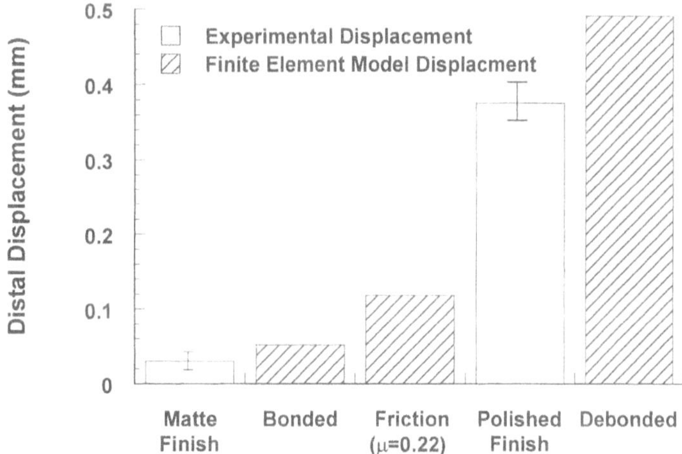

Fig. 4. Comparison of experimentally measured distal displacements of matte and polished surface finish stems to finite element predictions. (From Hustosky et al. 1999)

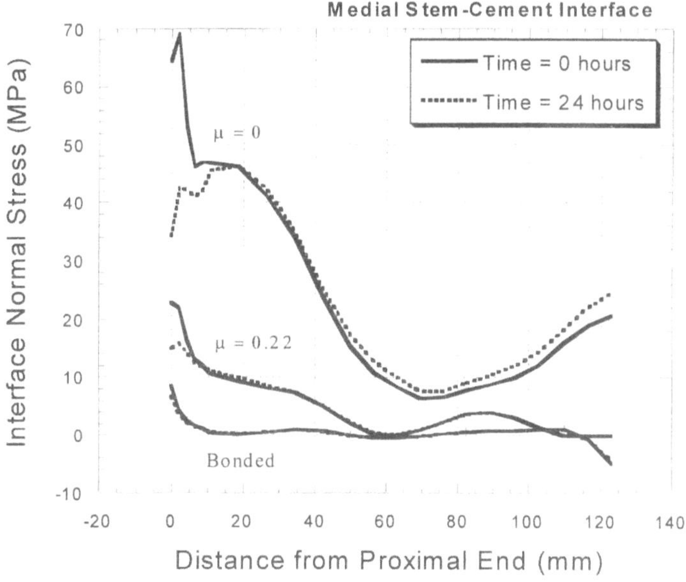

Fig. 5. Normal stem-cement interface stress distributions for the bonded, debonded with friction, and debonded without friction interface conditions initially and after 24 h of constant loading at the medial interface (Norman et al. 2001)

dence. The in vitro polished stem displacement occurs between a stem with friction and a stem without friction. Finite element results also show the medial stem-cement interface normal stress at time zero and after 24 h for bonded stem, for a debonded stem with stem-cement friction ($\mu = 0.22$), and for a debonded stem without friction (Fig. 5).

The normal stem-cement interface stress was greatest at the proximal medial region where the stem taper was the greatest. These normal contact pressures were also the greatest in the frictionless case and reduced significantly in the friction and bonded cases. The large normal contact stresses are indicative of "taper-lock" type fixation. The stress significantly reduced at the mid-stem and exhibited stress gradient-type appearances at the distal end of the cement mantle in the debonded without friction interface condition and the bonded interface condition to a lesser degree. The stresses were significantly smaller along the anterior, posterior, and lateral interface locations where the stem taper is small. A (viscoelastic) reduction in the normal interface stress occurred after 24 h of loading for all stem-cement interface conditions.

Discussion

The in vitro and finite element results presented were conducted for static loading with one cement and stem geometry. Other investigators have conducted additional experimental and finite element studies in this field (Harrigan and Harris 1991; Lee 1990; Lu and McKellop 1997; Mann et al. 1995; Chang et al. 1998; Miles 1990; Huiskes et al. 1998; Verdonschot and Huiskes 1998). Even given the limitations of this study, the general observations and conclusions are applicable to THR. It is known that bone cement creeps and that creep properties vary among the cements. We also know that creep is more likely to occur in debonded stems where the stem-cement interface stresses are higher. In bonded stems, the effect of creep is likely not important clinically because creep is small, less than 1% in laboratory tests. We also know that debonding of polished stems occurs at very low loads and that it increases with moisture sorption and mantle thickness (Gruen et al. 1999). Stems subside in vitro and exhibit a stick-slip phenomenon when the tip is unsupported, as otherwise end bearing occurs which would most likely reduce the amount of the distal displacement. We also showed that taper-lock does occur for static and dynamic loading in SLS and stair-climbing. All loading conditions provided a force necessary to produce a taper-lock equivalent to the original bond as confirmed by the pull-out test.

In conclusion, bone cement creeps and allows creep-induced subsidence. Creep of individual bone cements differs, and perhaps should be considered to optimize stem and cement selection.

References

Chang PB, Mann KA, Bartel DL (1998) Cemented femoral stem performance. Effects of proximal bonding, geometry and neck strength. Clin Orthop 355:57–69
Charnley J (1970) Acrylic cement in orthopedic surgery. Williams and Wilkins, Baltimore
Chwirut DJ (1984) Long term compressive creep deformation and damage in acrylic bone cement. J Biomed Mater Res 18:25–37

Gruen TA, Shockley D, Norman TL (1999) The effect of cement thickness and surface roughness on the strength of the metal-cement interface. 45th annual meeting, Orthopedic Research Society, Anaheim, CA, February 1–4, p 520

Harrigan TP, Harris WH (1991) A three dimensional non-linear finite element study of the effect of cement-prosthesis debonding in cemented femoral total hip components. J Biomech 24: 1047–1058

Harris WH (1992) Is it advantageous to strengthen the cement-metal interface and use a collar for cemented femoral components of total hip replacements. Clin Orthop 285:76–72

Huiskes R, Verdonschot N, Nivbrant B (1998) Migration, stem shape, and surface finish in cemented total hip arthroplasty. Clin Orthop 355:103–112

Hustosky KT, Norman TL, Kish VL, Blaha JD, Gruen TA (1996) The effects of creep on cement hoop stresses and axial displacement of a cemented femoral hip prosthesis in-vitro. Orthopaedic Research Society 42nd Annual Meeting, February, 1996

Hustosky KT, Norman TL, Kish VL, Gruen TA, Blaha JD (1998) Pull-out strength of a polished, tapered, cement total hip stem. Orthopaedic Research Society 44th annual meeting, March, 1998

Hustosky KT, Norman TL, Kish VL, Gruen TA, Blaha JD (1999) The effect of surface finish on the behavior of a tapered cement total hip stem. American Society of Biomechanics 23rd Annual Meeting, pp 136–137

Lee AJC (1990) Differential movement between implant and bone. In Older J (ed) Implant bone interface. Springer, Berlin Heidelberg New York, pp 131–135

Ling RSM (1992) The use of a collar and precoating on cemented femoral stems is unnecessary and detrimental. Clin Orthop 285:73–83

Lu Z, McKellop H (1997) Effect of cement creep on stem subsidence and stresses in the cement mantle of a total hip replacement. J Biomed Mater 34:221–226

Mann KA, Bartel TM, Wright TM, Burstein AH (1995) Coloumb frictional interfaces in modeling cemented total hip replacements: a more realistic model. J Biomech 28: 1067–1078

Miles AW (1990) A preliminary report on the stem-cement interface and its influence on the bone-cement interface. In Older J (ed) Implant bone interface. Springer, Berlin Heidelberg New York, pp 137–145

NIH Consensus Development Panel (1995) Total hip replacement, conference statement. J Am Med Assoc 273:1950–1956

Norman TL, Thyagarayan G, Sahgrama VC, Gruen TA, Blaha JD (2001) Stem surface roughness alters creep induced subsidence and 'taper-lock' in a cemented femoral hip prosthesis. In review, J Biomech

Norman TL, Kish V, Blaha JD, Gruen TA, Hustosky K (1995) Creep characteristics of hand- and vacuum-mixed acrylic bone cement at elevated stress levels. J Biomed Mater Res 29: 495–501

Norman TL, Williams M, Gruen TA, Blaha JD (1997) Influence of delayed injection time on the creep behavior of acrylic bone cement. J Biomed Mater Res 37:151–154

Norman TL, Gruen TA, Blaha JD (1999) Do all bone cements behave the same with regard to cemented stem fixation? Orthopedic Research Society 45th Annual Meeting, Anaheim, Calif., February 1–4, p 521

Older T (1997) Charnley low friction arthroplasty: a worldwide retrospective review at 15–20 years. American Academy of Orthopaedic Surgeons, 1997 Annual Meeting, paper no. 235

Saha S, Pal S (1984) Mechanical properties of bone cement: a review. J Biomed Mater Res 18: 435–462

Schreyer G (1972) Koinstruieren mit Kunststoffen. Carl Hanser, Munich, pp 502–569

Verdonschot N, Huiskes R (1998) Surface roughness of debonded straight-tapered stems in cemented THA reduces subsidence but not cement damage. Biomaterials 19:1773–1779

Subject Index